Feed Me!
I'm Yours

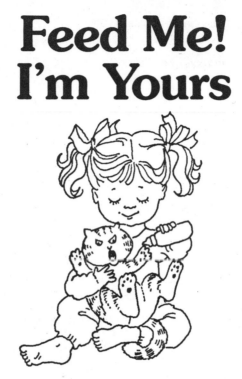

By Vicki Lansky

Illustrations by Kathy Rogers

D0596852

m Meadowbrook Press
Distributed by Simon & Schuster
New York

This book was first written in 1974 by six mothers, all members
of the Childbirth Education Association (CEA) of Minneapolis/St. Paul.
CEA is a nonprofit organization that prepares couples for a rewarding
childbirth experience.

Library of Congress Cataloging-in-Publication Data

Lansky, Vicki.
      Feed Me! I'm Yours / Vicki Lansky ; illustrations by Kathy Rogers.
  —Rev. ed.
    p. cm.
    Includes index.
    1. Children—Nutrition. 2. Infants—Nutrition. I. Title.
RJ206.L34 1994
649'.3—dc20   94-7354
                                                     CIP

ISBN 0-88166-208-9

Simon & Schuster Order # 0-671-884-433

First Printing, October, 1974
Updated Fourteenth Printing, July, 1978
Revised Edition, Twenty-ninth Printing, May, 1986
Revised Edition, Forty-first Printing, August, 1994

Editorial: Cathy Broberg, Craig Hansen,
and Jean D'Alessio, Christine Larsen, Sara Saetre
Managing Editor: Dale E. Howard
Production Manager: Amy Unger
Desktop Publishing: Jon C. Wright, Patrick Gross
Cover Design: Nancy Tuminelly
Assistant Art Director: Erik Broberg

Published by Meadowbrook, Inc.,
18318 Minnetonka Blvd., Deephaven, MN 55391

BOOK TRADE DISTRIBUTION by Simon & Schuster,
a division of
Simon and Schuster, Inc., 1230 Avenue of the Americas,
New York, NY 10020

99 98 97 96 95   45 44

Printed in the United States of America

Dedication

**To Parents Everywhere
from those of us who have been there
and
wish we knew then what we know now**

In the beginning, you'll be choosing between breastfeeding (the original health food) and formula, but at least these are two sides of the same coin—enriched milk. The field of food choices widens significantly by the time your child is six months old, and for the next number of years the responsibility for your child's food selection is mainly yours.

With this recipe book, we have tried to help you with that selection. Our recipes and ideas have been collected for their nutrition, convenience, and fun. We hope this effort will ease your task of meal preparation and help you enjoy your young infant, toddler, or preschooler while he or she is keeping you company at home.

Vicki Lansky
and Jill Jacobson
Stephanie Keane
Norine Larson
Mary Popehn
Lois Parker

Twenty Years Later—

In 1974 I was a young mother at home in suburban Minneapolis with two small children, ages one and three. I had majored in art history in college and worked as a sportswear buyer in New York City before getting married and starting a family. I had no experience with writing and publishing. But then I had an idea for a small cookbook that could be a fund-raiser for the local prepared-childbirth education group. With input and help from five other mothers, in a total of two group meetings (with at least a half-dozen children in tow at each meeting), I created a cookbook for new mothers. The only title ever suggested for the book was casually thrown out at one of those meetings—*FEED ME! I'M YOURS.* As they say, the rest is history.

The first hand-typed, hand-collated edition of *FEED ME! I'M YOURS,* with a black-and-white photo of my baby girl on its cover, was published in November 1974. The food editor of the Minneapolis paper gave us a wonderful review in the Sunday edition that Thanksgiving weekend, and we were flooded with orders. A few weeks later I remarked that many people were reordering additional copies. Suddenly my husband's ears perked up. Bruce realized that reorders were a different breed of sales from initial orders, and my evening project took on new interest to him. Within a few months we formed Meadowbrook Press (because we lived on Meadowbrook Lane), learned about typesetting and printing estimates, and became the publishers of *FEED ME! I'M YOURS.*

Over the course of the next year we learned how to publicize and market this new "infant" we had produced. Bruce convinced local media to interview me and local bookstores to buy the book. I went on television to demonstrate how easy it was to make baby food from scratch, taking time from madly invoicing and delivering copies of the book to those bookstores. We learned how to sell copies beyond Minneapolis. A successful strategy was our "relative marketing plan." We went to bookstores in markets where our relatives lived so we could afford to stay while we publicized the book.

Whatever we did seemed to work. It helped to be in the right place at the right time. Commercial baby food had been under attack, and I represented mothers at home who wanted alternatives that were easy and practical. We were forced to prove ourselves market by market, which we did. Today, morning talk TV is dominated by a handful of syndicated shows. This was not the case in the late seventies. Major cities had their own local talk shows that wanted the type of information I offered. To reach them, I was forced to travel and learn how to approach all the media. After we had sold over 100,000 copies of *FEED ME!* from our house, Bantam Books offered to publish a mass-market edition while allowing us to continue to publish our spiral edition. With their credibility behind us, Bruce was able to set up my appearance on the *Phil Donahue Show* (then broadcast out of Chicago) that boosted sales tremendously. (To get on the *Donahue Show* today, I think I'd need a book entitled *Sex and the Single Baby.*)

Counting our spiral edition and the Bantam mass-market edition, more than 3 million copies of *FEED ME! I'M YOURS* have been sold. I'm proud that *FEED ME! I'M YOURS* remains a valuable resource for parents. I have updated this new edition to be sure you benefit from new information, but it is still basically the same book that has served so many over the years. It has become a classic baby-food cookbook and one of the Horatio Alger success stories in the publishing community. It was my first book, and I thought my last. I was wrong. Another 24 followed. No one has been more amazed than I.

My two children, now in their twenties, have had the good grace to turn out well—*for there are no guarantees in this unique business of raising children*—for which I am grateful. Not only have they helped my credibility, but they have been a remarkable gift. They are my credentials, my graduate degree, as well as my pride and joy. They have even developed their own good eating habits which I will not presume to take all the credit for—only some of it.

—*Vicki Lansky*
Fall 1994

Contents

Introduction

Welcome to the world of the "haves"—people who have children, that is—and those umpteen new responsibilities, joys, anxieties, precious moments, and sleepless nights.

With your first child comes a new and demanding role: nurturing a totally dependent person. What you feed your child helps determine his or her mental and physical health. No one food contains all the nutrients we need, in the amounts we need, so we must opt for a variety of foods representing each of the four basic food groups. They are:

- Meat, fish, poultry, eggs and dry beans, and nuts
- Milk and dairy products
- Fruits and vegetables
- Breads, cereals, pasta, and rice

In the early 1990s, the U.S. Department of Agriculture developed a new way of looking at these food groups with what is called the Food Guide Pyramid. In addition to showing which different food groups we need to eat from, they added a new piece to the puzzle—quantity considerations. Fats, oils, and sweets are given a separate category. Fruits and vegetables, which used to constitute one group, are now divided into two groups, and everything is stacked with an eye to the proportional amounts we should eat daily.

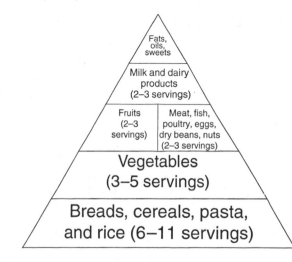

A good diet is one low in refined carbohydrates and refined sugars. Natural carbohydrates and sugars appear in fruits, flours, cereal, and vegetables. If your diet is varied and your quantity intakes are appropriate, your body will get what it needs.

Americans are often overfed but undernourished. The American diet contains far more calories than the body needs. The empty calories in foods made primarily of refined sugars squeeze the nutritious foods out of our diet. And even when we think we're watching our sugar intake, many of the grocery products we buy contain hidden sugars. Beware of what goes into those nice, consumer-oriented packages; read the labels of foods you buy. Let sugar be part of your family's balanced diet, but not the major part.

Nurturing includes providing a balanced and varied diet for your child, not determining the quantities he or she should eat. Children's appetites will change with their growth patterns. Each child's metabolism is different, with its own different food requirements. Your child will eat as much as his or her system demands at any time if you provide enough varied food at appropriate intervals. Only when your children are old enough to buy penny candy and junk food must you take care that nutritious foods aren't pushed out of their diet.

Your attitude toward food can encourage your child to develop a healthy attitude that can become a lifelong good habit. In fact, your attitude is the key to feeding this new child of yours.

**Be flexible. Respect strong food dislikes.
And remember,
Love is not equal to the amount of food
your child eats.**

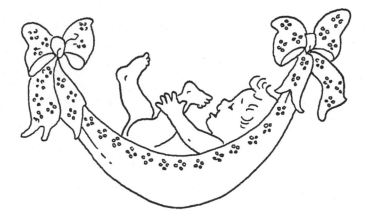

Baby Food

Economy, increased nutritional awareness, and a "back-to-nature" philosophy are some of the reasons why many parents are making their own baby food. Others discover that making baby food at home is much simpler and less time-consuming than they'd imagined. It can be gratifying to provide your infant with meals that save money (up to 50 percent), are free of additives and fillers, and are as fresh and nutritious as the foods you serve the rest of your family.

Homemade vs. Store-bought

You don't have to be a purist to make your own baby food. You probably won't stop using processed baby foods altogether, so when you purchase those little jars, read the labels carefully. Stay with the basic fruits, vegetables, and strained meats. Avoid combination and junior meals: you get less protein per serving in those than if you combined a jar of meat and a jar of vegetables yourself. Avoid jars containing sugar and modified starches as major ingredients. Forget the baby desserts; babies don't need them any more than we do.

Even store brands have begun responding to busy new parents' interest in better-for-you commercial baby food. In jars you can find *Earth's Best* brand baby food (for information call 800-442-4221). In your freezer section look for *Growing Healthy* frozen baby food, which is microwavable and packaged in single-serving plastic "trays." If it hasn't reached your freezer section yet, call them at 1-800-ABC-GROW for information. Yes, these baby foods cost a bit more, but they taste better, and you'll probably feel they are worth the cost.

Homemade Baby Food

After a ripe, mashed banana, probably the most commonly recommended first food is instant rice cereal. It has no allergic properties and is usually iron-fortified.

If you are nervous about making your own baby food, start with some of the many soft or pureed grocery-store foods available to you down the *other* aisles. These include unsweetened applesauce, canned pumpkin, banana (the riper it is, the more digestible it is), Cream of Rice cereal, and after about nine months, plain yogurt and cottage cheese (which may need a little extra mashing). A mashed baked potato (thinned with formula or breast milk) is also a fine first food.

When to Start

Don't be in a hurry to start your baby on solid foods. Milk (either mother's milk or formula) is a more important food than solids for the first half of your baby's first year. While the "breast is best," the American Academy of Pediatrics recommends that babies on formula drink an iron-fortified brand until they are twelve months old. Babies younger than one year get most of their vitamins and minerals from breast milk or formula. When solid foods are first introduced, they supplement, but don't replace, breast milk or formula.

For the full-term newborn, mother's milk or formula provides all the necessary nutrients. Even after the first four or five months of a baby's life, milk continues to be very important. Solid foods are often introduced at four, five, or six months. Some parents introduce a bit of cereal at bedtime on the

Microwaving Breast Milk, Formula, and Milk: Safety Tips

DON'T microwave frozen breast milk stored in a bottle. Instead, let the milk thaw by running lukewarm water over the bottle or setting the bottle in a pan of warm water. Reheating breast milk in a microwave is believed to reduce its anti-infective properties.

DON'T microwave formula in a glass bottle (as the glass could crack) or in colored plastic bottles (unless they are labeled microwave safe).

DO use clear plastic bottles—without bottle liners—when heating formula or milk. For a general guideline, heat a cold eight ounces on high for forty-five seconds. Leave the bottle uncovered in the microwave to allow heat to escape.

REMEMBER that microwave ovens can heat liquid unevenly, so invert (don't shake) a warmed bottle (with nipple replaced) about ten times to distribute heat, then test a few drops of the heated liquid on the back of your hand to check its temperature.

recommendation of a friend, relative, or pediatrician, to help a baby sleep through the night. There is no conclusive evidence from academic circles that this works—but there is no evidence that it doesn't work, either. We do know that an infant will not benefit nutritionally from cereal and that a baby's digestive track is usually not ready for cereals *or any solids* until four to six months of age. One pediatrician quoted in *Pediatric News* said, "My rule of thumb is to introduce cereal when a baby is taking five ounces of formula and is still acting hungry. If the mother thinks that it will help, then perhaps it will."

The introduction of solid food is a red-letter day in your child's life. He or she may not be grateful or even cooperative at first. Don't worry. Food is a great self-reinforcer.

If you find yourself spooning food into a mouth that is pushing the food back out, then your baby is still in the sucking-reflex stage and is not really ready for solid foods. Read this as a sign of what your baby's body is telling you, not as a rejection of your fine efforts. Don't be in a hurry. (Think of the time and money you'll save!)

On the other hand, if your baby is grabbing food off your plate, it's time to start new foods and textures. (Actually, you're probably a bit late.)

How to Start

Check with your doctor before trying new foods and introduce them to your baby one at a time, at four-to-five-day intervals, so you can detect the source of any allergic reaction. Offer new foods late in the morning or at midday, so you can monitor your baby's response during the afternoon and possibly avoid a sleepless night. A few spoonfuls at first will usually suffice. The idea is to introduce your baby to new tastes and textures—not to fill baby up. Signs of food intolerance include vomiting, gassiness, diarrhea, watery eyes, skin rash, or hives. Remember, three meals a day is an adult pattern for our culture, not a necessary approach for babies.

Two good bits of advice:

- **Follow your pediatrician's preference.** Babies prosper under as many different schedules as there are pediatricians. You also have to live with your pediatrician. (If you have definite opinions on the subject, check out several doctors' opinions before choosing one.)

- **Follow your own instincts.** Babies prosper under as many different schedules as there are parents. (If, on the other hand, your baby is not prospering, return to the previous paragraph.)

Whether you feed solids before or after breast or bottle depends on your baby's preference. Some babies need a little milk first, to take the edge off their hunger, so that they relax enough to be spoon-fed. Start by feeding solid foods once or twice a day, in the morning or evening. Choose a time when your baby seems hungry, is bored, or you both need a change of pace.

Allergy Alert

Many doctors recommend withholding egg white, citrus fruits, whole milk, and even some wheat products until a child is past one year of age, as they may cause allergic reactions, especially in food-sensitive families.

Something to Cook In

Clean pots and appliances are all you need for cooking your baby's foods. A crock pot, a pressure cooker, and a microwave oven can also be helpful. No, don't go out and buy them. Just use them if you have them.

Steaming fruits and vegetables is best because many nutrients are often lost in cooking water. Inexpensive steamer baskets that collapse to fit most pans work well, but make sure the pot you use has a tight-fitting lid to keep the steam in.

Cooking fruits and vegetables in a microwave is a form of steaming from the inside out and is an excellent way to cook small quantities quickly. As you add little or no water when cooking in a microwave oven, fewer nutrients are lost in the cooking process.

Something to Puree With

By pureeing the unseasoned food *you* eat, you will accustom your baby to the table foods he or she will eat soon.

Your fork can be used to puree, but some of the following might be more efficient:

- A **blender** can quickly and easily puree almost any food into the finest consistency. You will find that vegetables puree best in larger quantities and meats in smaller quantities. In general, you will be using the highest speeds to create a fine puree for the younger baby. As your baby grows, you can proceed to slower speeds for a coarser consistency. Blenders are reasonably priced and useful for making other child-oriented foods, such as shakes and homemade peanut butter. And you can also use a blender to reconstitute powdered milk or frozen orange-juice concentrate quickly. Pureed vegetables can be hidden in meat loaf or spaghetti sauce.

- A **food processor** can also be used to puree foods for baby. If you have one, wonderful, but if you don't, this use alone probably does not justify the expense of buying one. It is difficult to puree small amounts in a food processor, so be prepared to do large quantities and freeze most of it. (For information on freezing baby's food, see page 9.)

- A **standard food mill** can be purchased in a large or small size. You place food in the basket; as you turn the handle, the blade presses food through holes in the bottom of the basket. The food mill strains most cooked foods to a smooth consistency. Meat and poultry, however, will have a slightly coarser texture.

- A **baby food grinder** (a smaller version of the food mill) simplifies pureeing small amounts of fresh food for your baby. The food fits in a well; you place the turning disc on top. As you turn the handle and press down, the pureed food comes to the top and can be served right from the grinder. The grinder's small size makes it convenient to take along when you travel or eat out. It will grind fruits, vege-tables, and soft-cooked meats. The grinder conveniently sifts out the skins of peas and the hulls of corn.

After your baby outgrows the need for pureed food, you will find the grinder convenient for chopping nuts, grinding raisins and other dried fruits, softening butter or margarine, making egg salad, mashing a banana, mashing a baked or boiled potato, grating soft cheese, and probably many more uses.

Baby-food grinders are usually available in the baby departments of retail and discount stores.

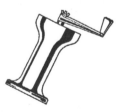

Handling and Storing Foods

Proper handling is important when you make your own baby food.

- Work with clean hands and clean utensils, *including clean grinders and cutting boards.*

- Prepare a food immediately after removing it from the refrigerator and freeze any leftovers or volume foods immediately.

You can store any open jars of commercial baby food in the refrigerator for two to three days. Commercial baby-food manufacturers do not recommend using the container as a serving dish because the baby's saliva on the spoon contaminates the food in the jar and speeds up the spoiling process. Another reason to avoid feeding a baby directly from the jar is the tendency to finish the jar and thus overfeed your baby. Plus, by transferring baby food from its jar to a serving dish, you can check the product for any foreign matter.

Freezer Options

When you make more food than your baby will eat in just one meal, you need a way to store the larger volume safely. Freezing your own foods gives you the variety and convenience of prepared foods. You will find it easy to cook in volume, and freezing quantities of food means you can always keep an adequate supply on hand and never need to rush to prepare food for a hungry baby.

You can easily freeze meal-sized portions for your baby using one of two methods: the "Food Cube" method and the "Plop" method. As your baby's appetite grows, you can add more "cubes" per meal or make bigger "plops." Before a meal, take out the food you want to serve. Thaw it in the refrigerator or warm it in a warming dish, microwave oven, or in an egg-poacher cup over boiling water. Remember that cold food and milk are acceptable to your baby, even if not to you. Their taste buds are not fully developed, so foods that seem warm to you may seem hot to your baby.

The "Food Cube" Method: Pour prepared, pureed food into plastic, pop-out ice-cube trays. Freeze immediately. Pop out the frozen cubes and transfer them to plastic freezer bags. Label and date. The food cubes can be stored for up to two months.

The "Plop" Method: Plop pureed or finely ground foods by the spoonful onto a cookie sheet. The size of each "plop" depends on how much you think the baby will eat at one meal. Freeze immediately. Transfer frozen "plops" to plastic bags. Label and date. "Plops" can be stored for up to two months.

A cube or a "plop" travels well for short journeys. By the time you've arrived, baby's meal is defrosted and ready to be eaten.

Food can also be frozen in empty, clean baby-food jars. Be careful not to fill them completely, because food will expand while freezing. Small Tupperware jars with lids can serve the same purpose. They stack easily in the freezer, too.

Keep protein foods, cereals, vegetables, and fruits in separate containers when freezing.

Baby's Cereals

Cereals are the typical first foods given to babies because they are fortified with an iron babies can absorb readily. You will find the commercial instant baby-cereals both convenient and nutritious. Rice cereal is commonly recommended first, since it is easy on most digestive tracts. But you can also easily make whole-grain and unprocessed cereals, such as Cream of Wheat, oatmeal, and Wheatena, by running them through your blender before cooking. It pays to make these cereals in quantity and freeze the balance by the methods previously described.

Hints: When preparing cereals for your baby, keep in mind that:

- A nursing mother may add expressed milk to cereals *or any foods* to make them more readily accepted, as the smell and taste are familiar to the baby.

- Any cereal can be sweetened with pureed fruits or a bit of brown sugar or molasses—*but avoid honey.* (See page 40.)

- A little plain yogurt (with active cultures) can be added to hot cereal. It gives a creamy texture to grainy cereals.

For cereal recipes, see pages 63–67.

Baby's Fruits

All fresh fruits, except bananas, must be cooked until they are soft—at least until your baby is about six to seven months old.

Canned fruits, packed in their own juice, are cooked in the canning process and are also easy to puree and serve. If they come in a sugar syrup, drain and rinse canned fruits before using them.

Bananas

Use one medium-size, fully ripe (speckled-skin) banana. Cut it in half and peel one half to use. Cover the remaining half (in the peel) and store it in the refrigerator for up to two days. Mash the half banana with a fork or put it through a baby-food grinder. The riper the banana, the more digestible it is for your baby. You can also peel ripe bananas, wrap them tightly in meal-size portions, and freeze. When ready to use, thaw and use immediately.

For a toddler who will accept chunkier foods, feed your child a banana right out of the peel with a spoon, one bite at a time.

Other Fruits

Apples, peaches, pears, plums, and apricots can be prepared by one of these methods.

Water Method: Wash fruit, peel, and cut into small pieces. Add 1/4 cup boiling water to 1 cup of fruit. Simmer until tender (10–20 minutes). Don't add sugar; babies prefer the natural sweetness of fruit. Blend or puree until smooth. Refrigerate what you will use that day and freeze the balance.

Steam Method: Wash fruit well, remove skin, and steam for 15–20 minutes. Cool. Remove pits. Blend or puree until smooth. Refrigerate what you will use that day and freeze the balance.

Microwave Method: Wash one piece of fruit. Remove core or pit. Place in a small glass with 2 3 tsp. water on the bottom. Cover dish lightly. Microwave 1 to 2 minutes until fruit is tender. Cool and remove skin. Mash or puree until smooth.

The following fruit-combination ideas are good for infants who have graduated to daily products or enjoy textures.

Tropical Treat

1/2 very ripe avocado, mashed or pureed
1/2 very ripe banana, mashed or pureed
1/4 cup cottage cheese or yogurt

Combine all ingredients.

Cottage-Cheese Fruit

1/2 cup cottage cheese
1/2 cup fresh fruit, raw or cooked
4 to 6 tablespoons orange juice

Blend quickly and serve cool.

Using this recipe, you can incorporate one of your prepared fruits into a whole meal.

Homemade Fruit Gelatin

Make your own fruit gelatin by dissolving **1 envelope unflavored gelatin** in **1/4 cup warm water.** Add **1 cup pureed fruit and chill.**

Baby's Vegetables

Fresh vegetables should be used whenever possible for best nutrition, flavor, and economy. Frozen vegetables are your best substitute for fresh. Canned vegetables, while not as nutritious, are still convenient and worthwhile; they are already cooked and need only be pureed. (Use the liquid from the can, if possible, because many nutrients are contained in it.)

Basic Vegetable Recipe

Cook beets, carrots, sweet potatoes, peas, green beans, and potatoes by one of these methods.

Water Method: Peel and slice for fast cooking or use frozen. Cook in 1 to 1-1/2 inches of water for 20 minutes. Puree or blend with some of the cooking water or orange juice.

Steam Method: Peel and slice for fast cooking or use frozen. Steam over boiling water until tender. Puree or blend, adding cooking water for right consistency.

Microwave Method: Cook a single item or a batch for pureeing and freezing. In a microwave-safe dish, with a touch of water, cook clean vegetables until tender. Potatoes need to be pierced several times first to allow interior steam build-up to escape. Single potatoes generally cook in 3–5 minutes.

Baked Sweet Potato and Apples

3/4 cup cooked sweet potato
1 cup applesauce or apples
1/4 cup liquid (milk, formula, or cooking water)

Preheat oven to 350°. Peel, core, and slice apples. Mix sweet potatoes and apples in buttered baking dish. Pour liquid over. Cover and bake for 30 minutes. Puree or mash with a fork.

Vegetable Soup

1/4 cup cooked pureed
vegetables
1 tablespoon butter or
margarine

1 tablespoon whole-wheat
or white flour
1/4 cup liquid (water or
broth)

Combine in a saucepan until warm.

Baby's Meats and Poultry

You can use any meat you have cooked for your family, or cook up to a month's supply of meat for your baby at a time, and puree it. If you want a smoother consistency, mix meat with a small, cooked serving of Cream of Rice and some milk and butter. Even a little water or juice will help pureeing in a blender. Combine chicken with a little banana and milk to get a smooth-textured meal. Meats cooked in a crock pot (minus seasonings) are tender and easy to puree.

All-Purpose Meat Stew

1/3 cup flour
1-1/2 pounds stew meat in
1-inch cubes
2 tablespoons oil
3 cups water

4 medium potatoes
5 medium carrots
1 package (10 ounce)
frozen peas

Coat meat with flour and brown in oil. Add water and cover pan tightly. Simmer 1-1/2 hours. Scrub, peel, and cube potatoes and carrots; add to meat. Simmer 15 minutes. Add peas and simmer 5 minutes. Take out a serving for the adults and puree the balance. Makes 4 to 5 cups.

Variation: Use any vegetable or 1/2 cup rice as a substitute for the potatoes.

Pineapple Chicken

Combine **boiled or baked chicken meat** in a blender with **canned, drained pineapple** that was packed in its own juice. For a snack drink, strain the drained juice, mix it with water, and serve.

Cockadoodle Stew

1 cup cubed chicken (or turkey), cooked	1/4 cup vegetables, cooked
1/4 cup rice, cooked	1/4 cup chicken broth
	1/4 cup milk

Blend or puree together and make into food cubes or "plops." (See Freezer Options under Handling and Storing Foods, page 9.)

Good substitutes for meat and poultry include cottage cheese, boneless fish, cheese, tofu, cooked egg yolks, macaroni and cheese, and (as your child matures) soft-cooked beans and nut butters.

Minimize Salt

These recipes do not require extra salt. Studies indicate that excess salt contributes to hypertension in later life. Since a taste for salty food is acquired, you can help your child avoid this health risk by minimizing salt in his or her diet.

Foods like rice pudding, chicken noodle soup, and even chunky applesauce can help ease a toddler into foods with more substance and texture.

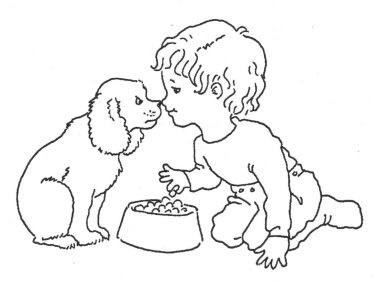

Finger Foods

Good health depends on sound eating habits. What your child eats, and how he or she eats, is established in the earliest years.

Introduce finger foods when your child's eye-hand coordination has matured enough so that he or she is able to pick up objects with fingers or a spoon and get them to his or her mouth. At approximately six to eight months, when your child is able to sit in a high chair and can reach for objects, a graham cracker, a few Cheerios, or a piece of soft cheese will be of great interest. If you allow your baby to experiment with food (despite the mess), you will have fewer problems in the long run. The more you allow your child to do, the faster your child will learn. Don't be surprised if you need two spoons for every meal–one for your child and one for you!

Be sure you have the proper equipment: a high chair, a spoon with a bowl small enough to fit the baby's mouth and a handle short enough for the baby to control, and an unbreakable cup with two handles and a weighted bottom (which may save you time cleaning up the floor). Speaking of floors, you may want to use newspapers or a plastic tablecloth under the high chair to save you the three-times-a-day cleanup.

A child needs far less food than many parents expect. A child eats when hungry and will take just what is needed to maintain the proper growth rate. Servings should be small, to avoid being discouraging; so should the plates or bowls. Better to serve small first and second portions than to be unhappy if a child has not finished a single large serving. Add new foods gradually. If your child should reject a particular food, return to a favorite and offer the new food again in a few days. It isn't always easy to respect your child's strong food dislikes, but it is important to try. Don't fret! Don't nag!

Sometime after one year of age, your child's appetite will decrease because the growth spurt of that first year slows down. Despite knowing this, it still comes as a surprise when children refuse to eat or finish foods they enjoyed or wolfed down just the week or month before. Toddlers change their food likes from day to day and meal to meal, so remember to offer old favorites and previously refused foods from time to time. Some children cling to the personal service of being fed, but ultimately (given the opportunity) they all learn to feed themselves.

Finger Foods *Not* Recommended for Babies Younger Than Twelve to Eighteen Months Old

Difficult to Digest	May Cause Gagging
Bacon rind	Hot dogs, whole or cut
Baked beans	in circle slices
Chocolate	Grapes, whole
Corn	Hard candies
Cucumbers	Ice cubes
Leafy vegetables	Nuts and raisins
Onion, uncooked	Olives
	Popcorn

Serve toast sticks, bread sticks, and raw carrot sticks to very young children with caution. Also, peanut butter should be used sparingly or thinned with milk for very young children so it will not stick in the back of the mouth and cause gagging.

Nuts and popcorn are *not* recommended, even for older toddlers! Some children are more susceptible to gagging than others, but all children have smaller air passages and weaker gag reflexes than adults.

Finger foods should be eaten only when your child is sitting up—not while running and not while lying down—and only when an adult is supervising.

Now that you know what specific finger foods to avoid or serve with care, here are several lists of ideas for foods that children *can* handle as they grow older.

Finger Foods Appropriate for Babies Six to Eight Months Old

Applesauce
Arrowroot cookies
Bananas, mashed or in small slices
Canned pears and peaches
Cheerios
Chicken liver and other tender meat, mashed or chopped
Cooked cereals
Cottage cheese
Graham crackers
Ground meat (which may or may not be accepted)
Potatoes, mashed
Pudding
Soda crackers
Soft-cooked vegetables, mashed

Finger Foods Appropriate for Babies Nine Months to One Year Old

Bagels, soft
Carrots and other vegetables, cooked soft
Cheeses, soft
Chicken, in soft-cooked pieces
Custards, soft
Eggs, boiled, scrambled, or poached (yolks only,
    if your child is sensitive or allergies run in your family)
Egg noodles
Fish, without bones (also gefilte fish)
French toast "fingers" (sliced in strips)
Macaroni and pastas (take advantage of interesting
    colors and shapes)

Meatballs, tiny ones
Meats, tender varieties of lamb, veal, and beef
Orange sections, peeled with loose membrane removed
Peaches, ripe and peeled
Rice
Spaghetti with meat sauce
Toast
Vanilla ice cream
Yogurt, frozen or regular

Texture becomes of great interest at this age. Most babies with two to four teeth are receptive to lumpier foods. Regardless of age, babies do not need teeth to chew; gums do an adequate job on soft foods. Chewier fruits and vegetables should be added as more teeth erupt. It is easy to drift into the habit of serving only soft fruits and vegetables, but it is wise to increase the chewy foods gradually as your baby's chewing ability increases.

Finger Foods Appropriate for Babies One Year and Older

Vegetables

Asparagus tips, cooked
Avocado, ripe
Broccoli florets, cooked
Carrot sticks, preferably soft-cooked or grated
Cauliflower, cooked
Celery, with all strands removed
Cherry tomatoes, halved
French fries
Green beans, cooked
Lettuce, shredded
Mushrooms, cooked
Peas, cooked
Pickle spears
Potatoes, mashed
Spaghetti squash
Sweet potato, cooked and mashed
Tomatoes, peeled

Fruit

Apples, peeled
Banana, whole or cut into sections
Blueberries
Cantaloupe, cut into bite-size pieces
Dried fruits (though avoid raisins for a while)
Fruit cocktail, canned
Grapes, halved for young toddlers
Kiwi pieces, peeled
Mandarin oranges, canned
Navel oranges, peeled and sectioned
Peaches, peeled
Pears, peeled
Strawberries, halved
Sweet cherries, pitted
Watermelon, pitted and cut into bite-size pieces

Hint: A toddler who won't touch fresh fruit may love dried fruits.

Dairy

Cottage cheese (add fresh or canned fruit for interest)
Deviled eggs made with mayonnaise
Hard-cooked eggs
Small squares of soft cheese, such as American or Gouda
Yogurt (may be served semi-frozen)
Grated or shredded cheese (can be purchased or homemade)

Yogurt

Yogurt is a good early baby food. It is creamy and easily digestible after your child is nine months of age. Yogurt with active cultures that break down the lactose should be the ones you choose.

Start with vanilla or plain yogurt. It can be used as a base for fruits (such as mashed banana) or cereals, or even those little jars of baby-food fruits. Yogurt can also be used instead of sour cream or buttermilk for cooking. Avoid fancy flavors and textured varieties for now.

Meats

Bacon, crisp*
Beef jerky*
Chicken or beef liver
Chicken or turkey, diced
Frankfurters, fresh*
Ham, cut into bite-size pieces*
Hamburger (try it in different shapes, such as sticks)
Lamb chops (with a bone that has no sharp points)
Luncheon meats*
Meatballs, small ones
Roasts, tender cuts (you may grind these)
Sausage*
Spareribs, well-cooked, little sauce
Tofu cubes
Tuna fish
Turkey, ground and cooked like hamburger
Veal

*These meats contain sodium nitrites that act as a preservative and coloring agent. They should be served in moderation. Some experts question the nutritional safety of nitrites, though amounts used in preservation have declined over the years. Of even greater concern is the large amount of fat and cholesterol these foods add to a child's diet.

Hot Dog Hint

Since hot dogs have been the most common cause of food-related choking among children younger than two years of age, monitor your child's consumption of them carefully. Better yet, slice a hot dog lengthwise (not in coin-shaped slices)—turn—and slice it lengthwise again, before serving alone or on a bun.

Breads, Cereals, and Other Grains

Arrowroot cookies
Bagels and cream cheese
Biscuits
Bran muffins (slightly frozen ones produce fewer crumbs)
Cereals, cold (dry or with milk)
Cereals, hot (regular or instant)
Graham crackers
Pasta, cooked (a variety of colors and shapes)
Oyster crackers
Pretzel rods (minus excess salt)
Saltines
Sandwiches, cut or broken into small pieces
Spaghetti, cooked
Toast, lightly buttered and cut into fourths
Triscuits
Zwieback

Pasta is a great favorite with tots. There is a wide variety to choose from today. The penne (tube) variety or the bow-ties are easier to eat than long strands of spaghetti. A child who disdains ground meat or spinach may just devour it when it is inside a ravioli square. It's easy to make even those long strands of spaghetti more feeder-friendly by criss-crossing a bowl of spaghetti with a pizza cutter to make smaller strands.

Avoid ready-to-eat cereals that are sugar-frosted, honey-coated, or chocolate-flavored. They add more unnecessary sugar to your child's diet and help create a sweet-tooth.

As your child's ability to use a spoon increases, so should the variety of bowl-type foods you serve. Be patient and try not to let the lack of neatness dissuade you from letting your child continue to practice.

Teething

This early-life passage may be quiet or traumatic. Try serving slightly stale, cold or frozen bagels, a frozen banana on a stick, the hard core of a pineapple, or a frozen food cube on a stick. Cold washcloths are good nonfood teethers. You can offer an ice cube served in a washcloth and held in place with a secure string or rubber band. Chilled pacifiers, teething rings, or even damp washcloths can be soothing, too. Some parents prefer toothbrushes, others offer rubber toys from pet stores.

Recipes for Teething Biscuits and Crackers

You can harden almost any bread by baking it at a very low temperature (150–200°) for 15–20 minutes. Your baby will enjoy teething on a variety of hard breads—such as whole-wheat and rye or pita bread, cut in strips—that you can make this way. But you may also like to try some of the following for economy and nutrition.

Hard, Round Teething Biscuits

2 eggs
1 cup sugar (white or brown)
2 to 2-1/2 cups flour (white, whole wheat, or a combination)

Break eggs into a bowl and stir until creamy. Add sugar and continue to stir. Gradually add enough flour to make a stiff dough. Roll out between two sheets of lightly floured wax paper to about 3/4-inch thickness.

Cut in round shapes. Place on a lightly greased cookie sheet. Let it stand overnight (10–12 hours).

Bake at 325° until browned and hard. This will make about twelve durable and almost crumb-free teething biscuits.

Banana Bread Sticks

1/4 cup brown sugar
1/2 cup oil
2 eggs
1 cup banana, mashed

1-3/4 cup flour (white, whole wheat, or a combination)
2 teaspoons baking powder
1/2 teaspoon baking soda

Combine ingredients and stir only until smooth. Pour into a greased loaf pan. Bake at 350° for about 1 hour or until firmly set. Cool, remove from pan, and cut into sticks. Spread sticks out on a cookie sheet and bake at 150° for 1 hour or longer, until the sticks are hard and crunchy. Store in a tightly covered container.

Oatmeal Crackers

3 cups oatmeal, uncooked
1 cup wheat germ
2 cups flour (white, whole
  wheat, or a combination)

3 tablespoons sugar
3/4 cup oil
1 cup water

Combine ingredients and roll onto two cookie sheets. Cut into squares. Bake at 300° for 30 minutes or until crisp. Be sure to roll thin and bake well.

Homemade Graham Crackers

1 cup flour (graham or
  whole wheat)
1 cup unbleached flour
1 teaspoon baking powder

1/4 cup margarine or butter
1/2 cup honey
1/4 cup milk

Combine flours and baking powder. Cut in butter or margarine until consistency of cornmeal. Stir in honey. Add milk to make a stiff dough.

Roll out on floured surface to 1/4-inch thickness. Cut into squares. Prick with a fork. Brush with milk.

Bake at 400° on an ungreased baking sheet for 18 minutes or until golden brown. If rolled thicker, these crackers can be used as teething biscuits, or use in Quick Graham-Cracker Dessert (see page 36).

For the Self-Feeder-Do-It-Yourselfer

While some little ones prefer the royal treatment of being fed, others prefer the independent route. Needless to say, encourage the latter. Here are some of the ways you can do this.

- Offer mashed potatoes. It adheres more easily to utensils.

- Serve a half banana *(not frozen)* on a wooden Popsicle stick or small plastic spoon.

- Mix dry cereal with yogurt or applesauce instead of with milk. It "holds" better to the spoon.

- Serve cereal in a handled mug, which is easier for a child to hold.

Finger Foods

- Serve finger foods in a paper lunch bag. Pulling edibles out of the bag turns mealtime into a game.

- Forget serving dishes, as they may prove to be a distraction. Pile food right on the high-chair tray.

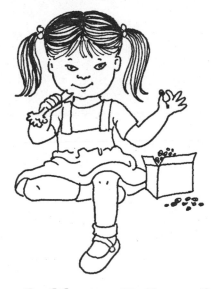

Toddler Meals

With your toddler now on table foods, you will probably notice that your meals are more often geared toward what your child will eat than the other way around. Save your gourmet delights for a few more years.

Although it may seem as if your child is growing like a weed, the truth is that he or she isn't growing nearly so fast as during the first year of life, when birth weight tripled and height almost doubled. That's why toddlers' calorie needs temporarily *decrease*—and why some are such finicky eaters. They simply aren't as hungry as they were as babies. In general, growth rates decelerate between eighteen and thirty-six months of age. Children at this age don't *need* a whole lot of food, so they often *are* picky about what they eat.

Don't let a finicky eater or child on a food jag throw you into a tailspin. Your goal isn't *to get* your child to eat—just *to let* your child eat. Hunger will out! Just be sure that what is eaten is not devoid of nutrients (such as filling up on soda pop) and don't worry about frequent snacks. Begin to look at them as minimeals.

Children have been known to survive by eating only peanut-butter-and-jelly sandwiches (or whatever) for extended periods of time. And never worry about one day's intake—or lack of intake. Small children only need a little meat to fulfill their daily recommended two ounces of protein. This is the equivalent of one chicken leg or a slice of luncheon meat.

Protein can be served in other, less obvious ways, too. Popovers (made of eggs and milk) or French Toast or Cottage-Cheese Pancakes (see page 59) are finger-friendly, high-protein meals. Quesadillas (cheese melted in a microwave on flour tortillas that are rolled up) are just another form of a grilled cheese sandwich. Egg-drop soup can be made by pouring and stirring quickly a beaten egg into any boiling chicken broth.

If you're simply out of ideas, you may want to consider some of the following. Try serving them on extra-thin bread or regular bread, sliced thin while partially frozen.

Lunch

Participation can be a great motivator. Playing "making-your-own-lunch" (or sandwich) often gets children to eat up their food. Have your children help you cut up green onions, parsley, lettuce, cheese slices, fruit, and similar foods, by using a scissors instead of a knife. Using a scissors helps to develop coordination and keeps kids busy for a *long* time.

Fill an empty ice-cube tray with finger foods such as fresh strawberries, cheese cubes, luncheon meat, hard-cooked egg wedges, and carrot sticks. Do this early in the day and refrigerate until serving time, when it will provide an interesting treat for some hard-to-please toddler.

Lunch Ideas

Deviled Ham—Spread on graham crackers or whole-wheat bread.

Cream Cheese—Spread on graham crackers. Very popular.

Egg Salad—Add mayonnaise for desired consistency. You may also wish to add finely chopped or grated celery.

Bagel Pizza—Top a bagel (or English muffin) with spaghetti sauce and shredded cheese, and broil.

Tuna Salad—Mash with a fork or put in a blender (depending on desired consistency). Mix with mayonnaise.

Lunch-in-a-Cone—Serve tuna salad, egg salad, yogurt, or cottage cheese in an ice-cream cone.

Full of Baloney—Fill slices of baloney with cottage cheese or spread with cream cheese and roll up. Secure with a toothpick.

Chicken Salad—Mix cubes of chicken with mayonnaise, finely chopped celery, and grated carrot.

Triangle Sandwiches—Spread whole-wheat bread with raspberry jam and top with thin slices of banana. Cut sandwich diagonally into fourths (to make triangles).

Cottage-Cheese Salad—Combine 1 can crushed pineapple, 1 cup cottage cheese, Dream Whip, and a 3-ounce package of (partially jelled) lime Jell-O mixed according to package directions. Set gelatin more quickly by substituting 1 cup ice cubes for 1 cup cold water. (If you don't have time to prepare the Jell-O, just sprinkle on part from the Jell-O envelope for color and flavor.)

French Toast—Substitute orange juice or condensed soup for the milk.

Leftover-Meat Sandwiches—Blend about 3/4 cup cubed meat, 1 hard-boiled egg, 1 tablespoon butter, and 1 tablespoon milk to make a paste. Keep in an airtight container in the refrigerator. (Pureed meat from baby-food jars can also be used as a sandwich spread.)

Grilled Cheese Sandwich—Place 1 to 2 pieces of American cheese between 2 slices of bread. Brown on both sides in 1 tablespoon margarine in a skillet.

Deviled Eggs—Add a face by using raisins for eyes, nose, and mouth.

Other Appealing Lunch Ideas

Peanut butter is a staple in most homes with young children. Purchase brands in the refrigerated section of your grocery store or those labeled "natural" where the oil has risen to the top, since the hydrogenated oil in the shelf-stable varieties is heavier and less healthy. Check the ingredients on shelf-stable brands, too.

A few additions to any common spreads can make sandwiches more imaginative and nutritious.

Peanut Butter:

- Peanut butter and ground raisins mixed with fruit juice
- Peanut butter and grated raw carrots
- Peanut butter topped with applesauce
- Peanut butter topped with artificial bacon bits plus honey
- Peanut butter and banana slices
- Peanut butter and cream cheese, blended with 2 table-spoons orange juice or honey

Cream Cheese and Others:

- Cream cheese with jelly
- Cream cheese with ground raisins
- Cream cheese with peeled and finely chopped (or grated) cucumber
- Chopped egg, cheese, and bacon bits
- Ground leftovers, eggs, and pickle relish
- Cottage cheese with grated pineapple
- Cottage cheese topped with sliced hard-boiled egg

Keep your sliced bread in the freezer. That keeps it from tearing when peanut butter or cream cheese is spread. Sliced bread, you will find, thaws in only a few minutes, so work quickly.

Pancakes are another excellent "bread" for sandwich spreads. Make (and freeze) extras the next time you're having them or buy the frozen variety. After applying spread, pop them in the microwave for 30–45 seconds before serving.

Homemade Alphabet Soup

1 teaspoon alphabet noodles	2/3 cup vegetable broth
2 teaspoons instant tapioca	a dash of salt
	a pat of butter

Cook over high heat for 3 minutes, stirring constantly. Remove from heat, stir in a dash of salt and a dot of butter.

Dinner

One of dinnertime's biggest problems is that your child's stomach is inevitably half-an-hour to an hour ahead of your meal schedule. You can feed your child early and avoid the next hour's headache. If you are determined that the whole family will eat together, offer a salad, side dish, or carrot as an appetizer. Sugarless gum or bubble gum may work to delay a hungry child. (Regarding gum, the concept of chewing instead of swallowing begins at about eighteen months, although your child will "lose" many pieces before the idea catches hold.)

For the younger set who are ready to eat corn-on-the-cob but not digest it, slice off the tops of the kernels, or slice down the middles of each row of kernels, so the corn can be sucked out.

And do you find that your child simply can't sit still during the meal? He or she must stand, bounce, climb, kick the table, go to the toilet, and generally drive you bananas. We can offer no remedy—only sympathy, for you are not alone. (We probably performed these same foul deeds as kids ourselves.)

Hint: An ice cube can bring many foods to an edible temperature quickly. Toddlers are not in favor of foods hot from the stove or oven.

Dinner Ideas

Tiny Meatballs—Add beaten eggs, oatmeal or wheat germ, and grated cheese.

Meat Loafies—Add ingredients above, but cook in a muffin tin. (Freezes well in this form. Reheat on a cookie sheet in oven or toaster oven.)

Macaroni and Cheese—Serve your combo or the grocer's. An all-time favorite.

Chicken Livers—Sauté in butter until tender; cut into pieces. Or wrap in bacon and broil.

Boned Fish—Use only fish that is quite fleshy, such as cod. Always check carefully for bones.

Corned Beef Hash—Place in a frying pan. Make a depression with the back of a spoon and break an egg into it. Cover and heat until egg has settled. Messy with fingers, but not bad with a spoon.

Pineapple Franks—Split frankfurters lengthwise and fill with drained pineapple; broil for 5–10 minutes. Older toddlers enjoy these.

Omelets—Whether your child likes omelets plain or with such additions as onions, green pepper, cheese, or wheat germ, cook them as large pancakes rather than scrambled. It's much easier for a child to eat omelets when they can be broken into pieces.

Dinner Recipes

Tuna Burgers

1 can (7 ounce) tuna, drained
2 tablespoons onion, chopped
2 tablespoons pickle, chopped
1/4 cup mayonnaise
slice of cheese, optional

Combine ingredients. Split and toast hamburger buns, and spread bottom half with tuna mixture. Top with a slice of cheese and broil for 4 minutes or until cheese melts. Add bun toppers.

Tuna Patties

2/3 cup Grape-Nuts cereal
1/2 cup milk
1 cup onion, finely chopped
2 tablespoons shortening
2 cans (7 ounces each) tuna, drained
2 eggs, slightly beaten
1 teaspoon lemon juice

Add cereal to milk; set aside. Sauté onions in 1 tablespoon shortening until tender but not browned. Add tuna, eggs, and lemon juice to cereal mixture. Blend thoroughly. Form 12 patties. Brown on both sides in 1 tablespoon shortening.

Salmon Soufflé

1 can (16 ounce) salmon
1 can (7-3/4 ounce)
   evaporated milk
3 tablespoons butter

3 tablespoons flour
1/2 teaspoon dry mustard
4 eggs, separated
paprika, optional

Drain salmon liquid into 8-ounce measuring cup and add enough milk to make 1 cup. Flake salmon and check for bones. In a saucepan, melt butter and blend in flour and dry mustard. Gradually add milk and cook, stirring until thickened. Remove from heat. Stir in beaten egg yolks and salmon; cool. Beat egg whites until stiff and fold into mixture. Pour into buttered 2-quart soufflé or casserole dish and bake at 350° for 45–50 minutes. Dust with paprika.

Loafer's Loaf

1 pound ground beef
1-1/4 cup uncooked
   oatmeal
1/4 cup minced onion
1/4 cup American cheese,
   grated

1/2 teaspoon celery salt
1 cup milk
2/3 cup tomatoes, chopped
1 egg, beaten

Combine all ingredients. Pack into greased loaf pan. Bake at 350° for 1 hour and 10 minutes. ("Uncooked" oatmeal is also known as "rolled oats" or "old fashioned" oatmeal—it's not the instant kind.)

Sloppy Poodles

1 pound lean ground beef
2 tablespoons flour
1 can (10 ounce)
   condensed French
   onion soup

6 hot-dog (or hamburger)
   buns

Brown meat in a large skillet and drain off excess fats. Sprinkle flour over meat and stir until flour disappears. Add can of undiluted soup. Simmer for a few minutes until mixture thickens and is hot. Serve on buns.

South-of-the-Border Casserole

1 can (15 ounce) chili
1 can (12 or 17 ounce) whole-kernel corn
1 package (8 ounce) grated cheese
1 to 2 cups nacho chips

Combine chili and corn in an oven or microwave-safe dish. Add grated cheese and then crumble chips. Press them down gently part way into the mixture. Bake in a 350° oven for 20 minutes or 5–8 minutes in a microwave oven.

Simple Soufflé

1/4 cup margarine or butter, melted
1/4 cup flour
1 cup milk

1 cup cheddar, Swiss, or mozzarella cheese, shredded (optional)
4 eggs
1/4 teaspoon cream of tartar

Melt margarine; stir in flour. Cook over medium heat until bubbly. Add milk and stir constantly until smooth and thickened. Add cheese if you are using it. Beat 2 egg yolks until smooth. Blend a little of the hot mixture into the yolk mixture. Return yolk mixture to saucepan and blend. Remove from heat. Pour into 1-1/2-quart casserole. Beat 4 egg whites until stiff, not dry, along with cream of tartar. Fold into casserole dish. Bake at 350° for 30–40 minutes. Delicious even when it falls.

Simpler Soufflé

1 can (10 ounce) condensed cheddar-cheese soup
6 eggs, yolks and whites whipped separately

Combine beaten egg yolks and cheese soup in a casserole dish. Fold in egg whites. Bake at 400° for 40 minutes or until done.

Orange Chicken

2 chicken legs and thighs
1/2 cup orange juice

2 tablespoons butter, melted
poultry seasoning

Place chicken in small baking dish and season. Mix melted butter with orange juice. Pour over chicken. Sprinkle with poultry seasoning. Bake 15 minutes at 350°. Turn and baste with juice mixture. Broil for 15 minutes or until chicken is crisp and tender.

Chicken Quiche

19-inch pie shell, unbaked
1/2 cup chicken, cooked
   and diced
1-1/2 cups Swiss cheese,
   shredded

3 eggs, slightly beaten
1-1/2 cups milk
2 tablespoons Parmesan
   cheese, grated

Place chicken in pie shell and add Swiss cheese. Combine eggs and milk. Pour over cheese. Sprinkle on Parmesan cheese. Bake at 375° for 30–35 minutes or until a knife inserted into center comes out clean. Allow to stand 10 minutes before serving.

Veggies

"If it's green, it must be yucky" is a philosophy you might run into (like a stone wall). Just increase the variety of fruits in your menus until your child's taste tolerance widens.

Some parents like to require their children to eat the same number of bites of vegetables as their own, individual ages. This adds pros and cons to being the oldest or the youngest child.

One way of introducing your child to a new vegetable, such as an artichoke, is by *not* serving it. "Adults-only" food often becomes more desirable when treated as forbidden fruit. You can "perhaps" let your child have a taste from your plate. Graduating to "adult" foods makes children feel more grown-up and at the very least saves you from throwing out or arguing over some tasty part of your meal.

Cooked Vegetable Tips

- Use up any leftover, cooked, yellow or white vegetable by mashing it, mixing it with an egg, and cooking it like a pancake or by baking it in a muffin tin.

- Sprinkle shredded cheese over each spoonful of cooked vegetables, or better yet, let your little cheese-lover do the job!

- Puree steamed vegetables and add to a simmering canned broth for a creamy soup.

- Have you tried spaghetti squash? This yellow, oval squash can be cooked whole in the microwave until soft. Cut it in half, remove the seeds, then use a fork to remove the pulp. It comes up like spaghetti strands. Serve with butter—or spaghetti sauce! A good, early finger food.

- Desperate? Try green noodles. They're made with spinach.

- Add moderate amounts of well-diced vegetables into a cheese omelet.

- Be creative. Artistic ideas with foods often create eaters. Use greens (broccoli, peas, and lettuce) as tree tops with pretzels for trunks. Half of a cherry tomato can be the center of a sun or a clown's nose; shredded carrot can look like hair.

- Hide pureed vegetables added in moderate amounts to meat loaf and spaghetti sauce. Hide a little puree under melted cheese on pizza or mix it with mashed potatoes. You might even want to try this in hamburgers. Experiment. Do it gradually.

- Mash some canned black beans into meat used for hamburger or meatballs.

- Offer pumpkin pie as yet another way to serve a cooked, yellow vegetable.

- Or make Sweet-Potato Chips. On a microwave-oven rack place 12 thin, unpeeled sweet-potato circle slices. Sprinkle with cinnamon-sugar and microwave 4–5 minutes until dry. Rotate during cooking. Let cool before eating.

Honeyed Carrots

3 tablespoons butter
4 cups carrots, sliced
3 tablespoons orange juice

1/4 teaspoon ginger
4 tablespoons honey

Combine all ingredients in a saucepan and cover. Cook over low heat for 30 minutes or until tender. Stir occasionally. Leftovers may be frozen.

Un"beet"able Gelatin

1 jar strained baby beets
1 package (3 ounce)
   strawberry Jell-O

cold water
1 cup boiling water

Chill strained beets thoroughly, then combine with cold water to make 1 cup liquid and set aside. Dissolve Jell-O in boiling water and add the liquid beet mixture. Chill until set.

Variation: Substitute cooked and pureed fresh or canned beets for baby-food jar equivalent. Beets vary, depending upon the season. If not sweet enough alone, add 1 teaspoon sugar to beet mixture.

Green-Bean Bake

2 packages whole green
   beans, frozen
1 cup sour cream
1/4 teaspoon pepper
   (optional)

2 tablespoons butter
1 garlic clove, sliced
   (optional)

Cook green beans with garlic, following label directions. Drain. Place in baking dish. Stir pepper into sour cream and spoon over beans. Melt butter in small saucepan. Add bread crumbs and toss. Sprinkle bread crumbs over sour cream. Bake at 350° for 20 minutes.

Raw Vegetables

Raw vegetables often meet with less resistance than those that are cooked. Combine this with the way your toddler attacks the hors d'oeuvres when your company is starting on cocktails and you have a fresh approach: serve raw vegetables with a dip.

Vegetables to serve children can include carrots, celery, cauliflower, radishes, cucumber spears, broccoli, sliced zucchini, slivers of green pepper, or mushrooms. The dip can have yogurt, sour cream, or cheese as a base.

Older toddlers are often fond of nibbling on frozen green peas straight from the freezer bag! Or try Chinese pea pods—they're sweet. Often, too, your children will eat vegetables they pick from your summer garden, while passing over the same item from your refrigerator.

Don't forget that, while not green, potatoes are an excellent vegetable. A baked potato, which takes only 3–4 minutes to cook in a microwave oven, can be a meal by itself, especially when topped with cheese, sour cream, spaghetti sauce, or anything your child loves. And of course it can be mashed, baked twice, and, yes, even fried!

Bunny Food

Combine **grated carrots** with **raisins**. Mix with some **mayonnaise**, or a bit of **honey** and **lemon juice**.

Pickled Carrots

For a new flavored snack, pack **carrot sticks** into finished pickle jars that still have liquid in them.

Quick Desserts

Quick Graham-Cracker Dessert

Crumble **1 graham cracker** into a bowl. Add **a teaspoonful of honey** and a bit of **warm milk**. Mash, mix, and serve.

Yogurt Sundae

Put some **yogurt (frozen or not)** in a dish. Add **fresh fruit** and pour **honey** over the fruit. Sprinkle with **granola, nuts, or wheat germ**. Top with a **maraschino cherry.**

No-Work Dessert

Serve any **fruit** with separate, small bowls of **sour cream** and **brown sugar.** Dip the fresh fruit into the brown sugar, then into the sour cream, and eat.

Chocolate Cream Cheese

1 tablespoon cream cheese   1/2 teaspoon sugar
1 teaspoon milk   1/8 teaspoon cocoa

Beat cheese with milk until smooth. Then beat in sugar and cocoa.

Apple Custard

1 apple
1 egg
2 tablespoons sugar

Preheat oven to 350°. Wash, peel, and core apple. Slice very thin and sprinkle with sugar. Beat the egg and fold into the apples. Put these into a well-buttered baking dish. Bake for 30 minutes.

Baked Banana

Peel firm **bananas** and place in a well-greased baking dish. Brush with **butter** and bake at 350° for 12–15 minutes. Remove from oven. With the tip of a spoon, make a shallow groove the length of the banana and fill with **honey.**

Banana and Apple Whip

1 small banana   1 teaspoon milk
1 small apple   1/4 teaspoon sugar

Wash, peel, and cut apple into small pieces (or grate it). Add the remaining ingredients and beat until blended. Serve immediately.

Banana Instant Pudding

2 ripe bananas, mashed
1/2 cup applesauce

2 tablespoons peanut butter
2 tablespoons honey

Stir until smooth, chill. Sprinkle with cinnamon or wheat germ before serving.

Homemade Fresh-Fruit Sherbet

1-1/4 cups fresh fruit
1 cup sugar
2 egg whites, beaten

Cut the fruit into small pieces. Mix the fruit and sugar well. Beat egg whites stiff and fold them in. Put in a freezer tray and freeze for about 2 hours, stirring occasionally. Cover with wax paper until ready to serve.

Chocolate "Ice Cream"

1/2 can sweetened condensed milk
1-1/2 tablespoons cocoa
1/2 cup regular milk

Combine ingredients and freeze for about 3 hours in a freezer tray.

Nutritious Frostings

Base:

2 tablespoons soft butter or margarine
1/4 cup honey
1 teaspoon vanilla

Cream together. For flavorings, add the following to the base and whip until smooth. *(Don't tell your children that the frosting is nutritious or they'll decide it's yucky before trying it.)* Use on breads and muffins, as well as on cookies and cakes.

Fruity Frosting

2 to 3 tablespoons fruit juice
1 cup nonfat dry milk
grated orange or lemon rind or chopped raisins or dates

Variation: You may substitute peanut butter for the butter or margarine in the base and add whatever else appeals to your family. Be sure to include the dry milk.

Spice Frosting

2 to 3 tablespoons milk, buttermilk, or yogurt
1 cup nonfat dry milk
dashes of cinnamon, nutmeg, and allspice

Banana Frosting

Mash one **banana** and add to **spice frosting.**

Chocolate or Carob Frosting

2 to 3 tablespoons milk, yogurt, or buttermilk
1/4 cup cocoa powder or carob powder
2/3 cup nonfat dry milk

More Frostings

- Sprinkle sugar and cinnamon on a cake or cookies just as you would on toast.

- Melt half a 6-ounce package of chocolate chips and half a cup of peanut butter, and spread over cookies or bars.

- Spread honey on cookies to make a good "glue" for adding candy decors, coconut, and other decorations.

- Dust confectioner's sugar on a cake or bar recipe for a completed look.

- Mix 1 tablespoon thawed orange-juice concentrate with 1 cup powdered sugar to make a "dribble" frosting.

Beverages

The following beverages make good meal supplements or snacks. Remember, though, that when your baby graduates to regular cow's milk, you should avoid serving skim milk until your child is at least two years old. Butterfats in regular milk are essential for growth and development in young children.

Hint: Extra formula, when baby graduates to milk, can be used for cooking, baking, or even in coffee.

Honey Alert

Avoid using honey and Karo-brand syrup in beverages and uncooked foods for infants younger than one year. There is concern that infants can't handle certain botulism spores. If these drinks aren't sweet enough with the pureed fruits, it's better to add sugar than honey.

Yogurt Milk Shake

1 cup vanilla yogurt
1 cup orange juice
1 ripe banana

Blend.

Tropical Blend

1/2 cup vanilla yogurt
1/2 cup crushed pineapple, undrained

1/4 cup orange juice
1/2 peeled Kiwi or banana

Blend. If too thick, add one to three ice cubes.

Sunny Sipper

1/2 cup orange juice
3 tablespoons lemon juice

1 can (13 ounce) evaporated milk
1 can (13 ounce) apricot nectar

Blend. Serve chilled.

Banana Smoothie

1-1/2 cups milk
1 large banana
1/4 teaspoon vanilla

Blend and serve at once. The banana you use can also be one that has been peeled and frozen, giving you a use for that last ripe banana.

Optional: For a new favorite flavor, add a tablespoon of peanut better when blending.

Triple Shake

1 cup each of three different fruits
5 ice cubes

Blend fruits and ice cubes in a blender for a thick fruit shake. Experiment with various fruits for favored combinations. This is also an excellent way to use up those last ripe pieces. Slice them up and freeze them in a plastic bag until you're ready to combine with others.

Sangria Junior

1 small bottle white grape juice or cranberry juice
1 cup orange juice
1 cup sliced grapes

1 cup sliced-in half orange circles
1 cup cleaned and sliced strawberries, kiwis, or peaches

Serve with swizzle sticks or long forks and a straw.

Milk Eggnog

1 cup cold milk
1 egg

1/4 teaspoon vanilla
1 tablespoon honey
nonfat dry milk (optional)

Blend. Eggnog is another way of providing a good protein for your older toddler who has decided to abstain from most of the protein foods you are offering. Fortify with several tablespoons nonfat dry milk if you wish.

Variation: Orange juice may be substituted for the milk.

Egg Alert

Some of these drink recipes call for raw eggs, which is a good way of serving eggs to those children for whom "egg" means "Forget it!" Most physicians don't recommend serving egg (cooked or raw) to babies under six months or even to babies under one year, since some infants have an allergic reaction to egg white. Try using the yolk initially, and freeze the whites for later use in baking.

Because raw eggs (the shells, actually) can be a carrier of the bacteria salmonella, they are not a good choice for infants younger than nine to twelve months old. Their stomachs are much too sensitive to the effects of this bacteria.

Orange Delight

1 to 2 eggs
1/3 cup orange-juice concentrate
1/4 cup nonfat dry milk
1/2 banana (or equivalent fruit)
3/4 cup water
ice

Mix in blender. The more ice you add, the slushier the drink becomes.

Water

The beverages given above are great snacks, but kids also need to drink to satisfy their thirst and the body's need for fluids. Water is still the best (and cheapest) thirst quencher. Make drinking it an early habit. Sometimes kids need to have water's appeal reinforced by fun containers (a biker's bottle, a canteen, or a new plastic cup). Keeping water cold also adds to its acceptance.

Juices you buy (labeled *100% real fruit juice* on their containers), not juice drinks, are also good beverage choices. Be aware that apple juice in large amounts actually can contribute to chronic diarrhea in young children. You may wish to water it down if you have a real "apple-juice-only" lover. Avoid sodas as a staple—especially those high in caffeine, such as colas and chocolate-flavored or some orange-flavored sodas.

For the same reason, go easy on ice tea. Many doctors recommend waiting until your child is one year of age before introducing orange juice, owing to its high acid content.

Milk

After water, your next best beverage for kids is whole milk. Sixteen to twenty-four ounces of milk a day is plenty for a toddler. And toddlers who eat yogurt, cheese, and other dairy products can get by with lots less. Don't move on to skim milk until your child is four to six years of age or your doctor recommends a change. Here are some ways to add interest to this staple.

Milk Marvels

Add one of the following to 1 cup cold milk for nutrition and interest. Mix well in a blender.

- 1/2 banana, mashed or frozen

- 1 scoop of fruit-flavored ice cream or sherbet

- 1/2 cup frozen strawberries plus the syrup, or 1/2 cup fresh berries plus some sweetener, if needed

- 1/2 cup of any fresh, bruised berries; 2 tablespoons sugar; 1 tablespoon lemon or orange juice

- 1/2 banana, a scoop of vanilla ice cream, and 1 tablespoon chocolate syrup

- canned peaches or pears, 2 tablespoons fruit syrup, and 1 scoop vanilla ice cream

To a mug of hot cocoa and milk, add a spoonful of creamy peanut butter and a dash of whipped cream.

Fortified Milk

The protein value of milk can be increased by adding some nonfat dry milk to regular milk. But do so only in moderation, especially if your child already has a low fluid intake. *Never give a calcium supplement without professional advice, however.*

Hint: For the child who refuses milk, remember that it can be "eaten" in the form of puddings, custards, cheese, yogurt, or creamy soups.

Hints for the do-it-yourself (at last!) drinker:

- Fill a glass only about 1/3 full to limit waste when the inevitable spills occur. Provide refills when requested.

- Have your child practice drinking water from a cup while he or she is taking a bath.

- Cut straws down to size for the child and the cup or glass being used.

If Your Child Can't Drink Milk

Milk intolerance is a common problem that defies the slogan "Milk Is for Everybody." It is not. Actually, the majority of the world's population cannot tolerate cow's milk. Most able are those of Western European descent, and even among this group, a significant percentage (20%) can't tolerate milk. Symptoms such as abdominal pain, bloating, gas, diarrhea, or nausea may well be related to the ingestion of cow's milk.

This intolerance, referred to as "lactose intolerance," results from an inability to digest the natural sugar in milk. An enzyme ("lactase") in the intestinal lining breaks down lactose (milk sugar) into simple, digestible sugars. When lactase is completely absent (a rare condition) or present in low concentrations (which is more common), consumption of milk products may cause discomfort. In a young child, an intestinal infection can cause temporary reduction of lactase. (This is one reason why doctors eliminate milk when a child has diarrhea.)

The amount of milk tolerable to those with lactose intolerance varies with the level of lactase in the intestine. For example, some persons who cannot digest moderate amounts of milk can tolerate yogurt or aged cheeses.

The words on labels to watch for are: milk (condensed, evaporated, fresh, whole, skim), buttermilk, sweet or sour cream, malted milk, lactose, nonfat dry milk solids, curds, whey, margarine, butter, sodium caseinate, casein, and lactalbumin. (The last three are additives made from the protein of cow's milk and are permissible for those who cannot tolerate lactose—milk sugar—but not for those who are allergic to milk.)

In addition to the obvious labels to read, if your child has milk intolerance, you must read the product labels of items such as frozen fish sticks, frozen egg substitutes, dry cereals, salad dressing (when cheese has been added), gravies, and vitamin capsules and medications using lactose fillers.

Cooking Milk-Free

In cooking, you can often substitute another liquid for milk. When a recipe calls for milk or cream, try water, chicken stock, beef stock, wine, or fruit juices. Orange and apple juice—even 7-Up—work nicely in many recipes for baked products. With a bit of experimenting, you'll find substitutes of your own that work.

Soy powered milk, available in health-food stores, supermarkets, and drug stores, can be reconstituted and used. Some nondairy coffee lighteners are useful, but be sure the one you select omits lactose. Infant soy formula may be palatable in some recipes or used on cereals.

Or maybe you've discovered Lactaid milk or Lactaid-brand caplets. This supplement helps restore the enzyme in the body that makes dairy foods more digestible. For a free sample or information, call 1-800-LACTAID. Another similar product on the market is called Dairy Ease.

Puddle Cake

1-1/2 cups flour (white or half white, half whole-wheat)	3 tablespoons cocoa or carob powder
1 cup sugar	1 teaspoon vanilla
1 teaspoon baking soda	1 teaspoon vinegar
	6 tablespoons cooking oil
	1 cup water

This classic dessert is also milk-free.

Sift flour, sugar, soda, and cocoa into an ungreased 8 x 10-inch cake pan. With a mixing spoon, make three holes in the dry mixture. Place vanilla in the first hole, vinegar in the second, and oil in the third. Pour water over all and stir with a fork to moisten dry ingredients. Do not beat. Bake at 350° for 35 minutes.

For more recipes, check out my *Taming of the C.A.N.D.Y. Monster* cookbook (Book Peddlers).

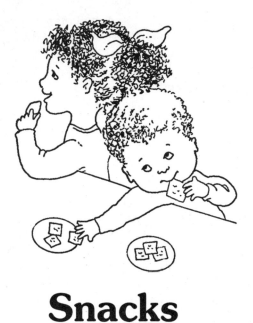

Snacks

Snacking is a way of life in most American households. It need not be a dirty word—nor need it be on junk! Junky snacks push the nutritious foods out of our diet, contribute to tooth decay, and add pounds. But nutritious snacks should be considered part of your child's overall nutrition for the day.

We snack on what is handy. Having wholesome snacks on hand—bought or made—is part of our job. Fruits and vegetables are the most obvious nutritious snack foods, plus most of the finger foods listed in the previous chapters.

Crackers are lower in sugar than cookies. Many are now available in reduced-salt versions. And don't forget lightly buttered whole-grain toast. Toast can be made more interesting by buttering bread lightly or sprinkling it with a little cinnamon and sugar, or Parmesan cheese, before cutting it with cookie cutters. (You can use just one shape at a time for a theme, such as a fish-shaped cookie cutter for a "fishy" snack.) Place shapes on a cookie sheet and toast slightly in an oven at 350°.

Spread mashed bananas (or any other favored spread) on mini-rice cakes for a nice snack.

Raisins and other dried fruits have fallen from favor in the dental community because they consist of sugars, albeit natural, that stick between teeth and promote tooth decay. Consider moving dried fruits from snacktime into the main mealtime.

And don't rule out cold, cooked pastas. Elbow macaroni by itself or served with grated cheese also makes a good snack food.

Finger Jell-O

2 envelopes unflavored gelatin
2-1/2 cups water
1 package (6 ounce) or 2 packages (3 ounce) Jell-O

It disappears before your very eyes! Dissolve unflavored gelatin in 1 cup of cold water. Set aside. In a saucepan, bring 1 cup of water to a boil and add Jell-O. Bring to a boil again, then remove from heat. Add gelatin mixture. Stir and add 1/2 cup cold water. Pour into a lightly greased pan and refrigerate until firm (about 2 hours). Cut into squares (or use a cookie cutter) and store in an airtight container in the refrigerator.

Or avoid using commercial Jell-O altogether by combining 3 envelopes of unflavored gelatin with one 12-ounce can of frozen juice concentrate and 12 ounces of water. Soften the gelatin in the thawed juice and bring the water to a boil. Add the juice-and-gelatin mixture to the boiling water and stir until gelatin dissolves. If the juice needs extra sweetening, add it here. Follow directions for chilling as in above recipe.

Jell-O Pizza

Mix above recipe for Finger Jell-O using **lemon- or orange-flavored gelatin.** Pour in just enough to fill a lightly greased pizza pan to the edges and chill in refrigerator until firm. (Chill balance of Jell-O in a second pizza pan or another container.) Spread the firm Jell-O lightly with **vanilla yogurt or whipped cream.** Sprinkle on a topping of **sliced fruits** (such as kiwis, bananas, or strawberries). Cut into wedges and serve.

Apples in Hand

Peel (optional) and core **a whole apple**. Mix **peanut butter** with one of the following: **raisins, wheat germ, or granola.** Stuff this mixture into the hole of the cored apple. Slice in half to serve. Or stick the apple half on a Popsicle stick. It's both novel and neat that way.

Stuffed Celery

Stuff **celery sticks** with **cream cheese or peanut butter. Raisins** may be added on top of the spread. Depending on the age and chewing ability of the child, you may want to remove the strands from the celery.

Turn a stuffed celery stick into a "racing car" by pushing a toothpick through each end of the celery piece and attaching a single grape to the exposed toothpick ends for "wheels." *But make sure your child doesn't eat the toothpicks!*

Grinder Snacks

Grind **figs, dates, and raisins** in equal amounts. (Nutmeats, too, if you wish.) Add a small amount of **lemon juice** to **a cup of graham-cracker crumbs**. Make small balls out of your ground mixture and roll in crumbs for coating. (Your baby-food grinder can come in handy here.)

Peanut-Butter Roll-Ups

1 container peanut butter
4 slices bread
Honey or jam (optional)

Cut away the crusts from the bread slices. Place each slice on a hard surface and use a rolling pin to roll it flat. With a knife spread a thin layer of peanut butter on the flattened bread. Spread jam or drizzle honey onto peanut butter. Roll each piece of bread up jelly-roll style. Slice roll into one-inch pieces and secure with toothpicks.

Peanut-Butter Balls

1/2 cup peanut butter
3-1/2 tablespoons nonfat dry milk
a bit of honey
optional: raisins, nuts, coconut, wheat germ, sunflower
    seeds, and brown sugar

Combine ingredients, roll into balls, and store in refrigerator.

Goodie Balls

1/2 cup peanut butter
1/2 cup honey
1/2 cup instant cocoa or
    carob powder

1 cup peanuts or soy nuts
1/2 cup sunflower seeds
1 cup toasted wheat germ
dry coconut flakes

Combine first six ingredients. Roll into balls and roll in
coconut. Refrigerate if using a refrigerated brand of peanut
butter, which is preferable.

Chocolate Peanut-Butter Sticks

8 ounces semisweet
    chocolate
6 tablespoons peanut butter

1 teaspoon vanilla
1 cup toasted wheat germ

Melt chocolate and blend with peanut butter and vanilla. Stir in
wheat germ. Press into a buttered 8-inch-square pan and chill
until firm. Cut into bars and store in a container in the refrigerator.

Cheesy Wheats

4 cups spoon-size shredded wheat
1/2 cup margarine
1 cup cheese, shredded

In a large saucepan, melt margarine. Add cheese. When the
cheese begins to melt, add shredded wheat. Toss to coat well.
Refrigerate if not to be eaten within an hour or two. (This recipe
can be easily adapted for a microwave oven.)

Cereal Sticks

1/2 cup butter or margarine
1 cup sugar
2 eggs
1 teaspoon vanilla
2-1/2 cups flour (white,
    whole wheat, or a
    combination)

1/4 teaspoon baking soda
1/2 cup plus of cereal (such
    as Grape-Nuts, granola,
    or wheat germ)

Blend together the first six ingredients, plus 1/4 cup of the cereal. If the dough is too soft, add more flour. Roll a small piece of dough into a stick, and then roll the stick in the extra cereal to coat. (Employ anyone in your family who's experienced with play dough.) Place on a lightly greased cookie sheet and bake at 400° for 8 minutes or until slightly browned.

Uncandy Bars

1 loaf of bread (white, whole
    wheat, or other)
1 package peanuts,
    chopped

1 cup peanut butter
peanut oil
1/4 cup toasted wheat germ
    (optional)

Trim the crust from the bread. Cut bread slices in half. Put bread and crusts on a cookie sheet in the oven overnight, until dry, or place in a 150° oven for 1/2 hour or until dry. Put only the dried crusts in a blender until finely crumbed. Combine crumbs with chopped nuts. Add wheat germ, if desired. Thin the peanut butter with oil. Spread or dip the bread slices in the peanut butter, then roll them in the nut-and-crumb mixture. Dry them on a cookie sheet. Store in an airtight container. No need to refrigerate if you are using shelf-stable peanut butter.

Variation: If candy isn't candy to you without chocolate, add 1 tablespoon instant cocoa to the thinned peanut butter.

Oatmeal Bars

2 cups oatmeal, uncooked   3/4 cup brown sugar
1/2 cup butter or margarine   dash of baking soda

Boil sugar, shortening, and baking soda. Add oatmeal. Blend. Spread mixture in a well-greased 8-inch-square pan and bake at 350° for 10 minutes. Cut into bars while warm.

Bite-of-Apple Cookies

1/2 cup margarine   1/2 teaspoon cinnamon
1 cup brown sugar   3/4 cup wheat germ
2 eggs   1 cup apples, peeled,
1-1/2 cups flour   cored, and finely
1/2 cup oatmeal, uncooked   chopped
2 teaspoons baking soda

Cream margarine, sugar, and eggs. Mix dry ingredients and combine with creamed mixture. Add apples. Drop spoonfuls onto a greased cookie sheet. Bake at 350° for 10–15 minutes.

Super Cookies

1-1/2 cups oatmeal,   1 teaspoon cinnamon
   uncooked (or Swiss   1/3 teaspoon cloves
   Familia)   1/2 cup oil or butter, melted
1/2 cup nonfat dry milk   2 eggs, beaten
1/2 cup wheat germ
3/4 cup sugar (or 1/2 cup
   honey)

Mix dry ingredients. Add melted butter and beaten eggs. Spoon onto greased baking sheet. Bake at 350° for 12–15 minutes.

Note: "Uncooked" oatmeal is also known as "rolled oats" or "old fashioned" oatmeal—it's not the instant kind.

Nutritious Brownies

1/4 cup vegetable oil
1 tablespoon molasses
1 cup brown sugar
2 teaspoons vanilla
2 eggs
1/2 cup pecans or walnuts, broken

1 cup wheat germ
2/3 cup nonfat dry milk
1/2 teaspoon baking powder
1/4 cup dry cocoa or 2 squares unsweetened baking chocolate

Mix together the first seven ingredients. (If using squares of chocolate, melt in a double boiler and add here.) Sift the dry milk, baking powder, and cocoa through a sieve into the other ingredients and stir well. Spread in a heavily greased 8-inch-square pan and bake at 350° for approximately 30 minutes. Turn out of pan immediately and cut into bars while still warm.

Fruit Roll

Use apples, peaches, pears, nectarines, or canned pumpkin to make this yummy dried "candy." The fruit can be the "too-hard-to-eat" variety or the "too-ripe-and-the-last-piece" variety. It may even be well-drained, canned fruit. Mash or puree the fruit. Two methods work well:

Blender method: Peel and core fruit, blend until smooth, and then cook five minutes in a saucepan over moderate heat.

Freeze-defrost method: In advance, peel and core fruit, wrap and freeze. Remove from freezer an hour before using so fruit can begin to defrost. Cook in a saucepan, mashing with a fork as you go, for 5–10 minutes. If the fruit is very watery, drain it.

While cooking, add 1 teaspoon honey for each piece of fruit you are using. (Cook different fruits separately, though you can cook one piece or a dozen of the same type at once.)

Lay out clear plastic wrap (or cut open small plastic bags) on cookie sheet or broiling tray. Use one piece of plastic for each piece of fruit you have cooked. Spoon mixture onto the wrap, staying away from its edge. Spread as thin as possible. Spread another piece of plastic wrap over the mixture and press down with a wide spatula to make evenly thin. Remove this top sheet of plastic before drying.

Turn oven to its lowest possible heat or just use the pilot light. Place tray in the oven and leave overnight (6–8 hours). The plastic wrap will not melt! If the fruit is dry by breakfast, remove from the oven. (If not, wait a while longer.) Roll up the plastic wrap (with the dried fruit) as if it were a jelly roll.

Then peel and eat!

The rolls will last several months this way—if your children don't discover them, that is. If you don't understand how this should look, stop in at a health-food store and ask to look at their fruit rolls. And notice the price!

Variation: Core and peel an apple. Slice it into thin rings and dry as for fruit roll.

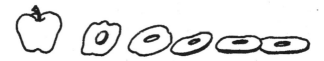

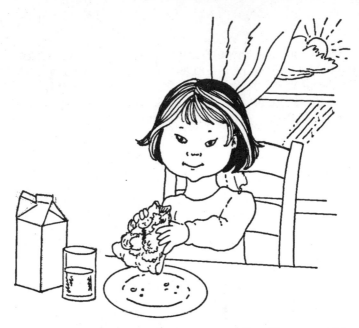

Pizza for Breakfast?

It's 7:45 in the morning. Your husband needs to leave for work by 8:15, and he's in the kitchen frying some eggs. You're giving milk to your three-month-old, and your three-year-old, Chris, doesn't want any old fried eggs. He'd rather have leftover pizza for breakfast. Dad says, "No, pizza isn't breakfast food. Here's a nice piece of toast with jelly." You finish feeding and changing baby, give Chris some cold cereal with milk and sugar, plus a glass of orange juice, and then relax with a cup of coffee or tea. You guess you'll have something to eat around 10 a.m. Sound familiar?

No one wants to be creative at 7 a.m., but breakfast is a very important meal. And it's important for you to be as good a model as possible for your kids in this area as well as in other aspects of your life. People who skip breakfast are more likely to eat between meals and often consume more calories in a day than people who eat breakfast. If your children see you eat a well-balanced breakfast, they will probably develop good eating habits, too.

Part of the problem stems from our stereotyped ideas of breakfast food, as just illustrated. Maybe now is the time to change our stereotypes about mealtime menus. A peanut-butter sandwich, a hunk of cheese and whole-wheat toast, or a container of yogurt are perfectly acceptable breakfast foods.

Leftovers have traditionally been served at lunch and dinner. Just for variation, why not serve leftover pizza, hamburger, casseroles, chops, or spaghetti for breakfast? And save eggs, cereal, or something "breakfasty" for the noon or evening meal? In a lot of cases, you don't even have to warm up the leftovers!

The following recipes and ideas are aimed, to a great extent, toward making breakfast enjoyable and nutritious, not only for your kids, but for your entire family.

Breakfast Pizza

In case you have leftover spaghetti sauce, here's a good way to use it up!

spaghetti sauce
English muffins
butter or margarine
cheese (such as mozzarella, cheddar, American, or Colby)

Split muffin and toast lightly. Spread with a little butter or margarine and top with 1 to 2 tablespoons spaghetti sauce. You may add bacon bits, mushrooms, or anything else you want. Then lay a couple of slices of cheese on the top. Heat muffin pizza under the broiler until the cheese is gooey (3–5 minutes).

Other nontraditional possibilities for breakfast

- Grilled (or ungrilled) cheese sandwiches
- Cottage cheese
- Soup and cheese
- Eggnog drinks (see page 41)

Eggs

Eggs are a traditional part of the breakfast scene; some kids really go for them and others don't. Eggs are also good dinner fare. Here are a few ideas that may not convert the egg-haters but that might lure the "not-so-crazy-about-eggs" bunch!

Bull's Eye

1 egg
1 slice bread
margarine or butter

Use a 2-inch-round cookie cutter to cut out the center of the bread. Spread margarine generously on both sides of the remaining bread. Brown one side of the bread in a moderately hot, greased frying pan, and then turn over. Crack the egg into the hole in the bread and cook until the white is set. You may need to cover the pan to help the egg white set quickly. Lift out carefully and serve.

You may wish to use a cookie cutter shaped as a heart for Valentine's Day, a bunny for Easter, and a bell for Christmas.

Peanut-Butter Custard

1-1/3 cups milk
1/3 cup nonfat dry milk
1/3 cup peanut butter

2 eggs, beaten
3 tablespoons honey

Warm the liquid milk; stir in dry milk and blend with peanut butter until smooth. Mix in the eggs and honey, and pour into greased custard cups. Set the cups in a pan of hot water (water should come up to the same level as the custard). Bake at 325° for 30 minutes or until a knife inserted in the center comes out clean. Refrigerate and serve cold.

Bread Omelet

2 tablespoons bread
  crumbs
2 tablespoons milk

1 egg, separated
1/2 teaspoon butter or
  margarine

Mix the bread crumbs and milk. Soak for 15 minutes or overnight in a covered bowl in the refrigerator. In another bowl, beat the egg yolk well. In a third bowl, beat the egg white until stiff but not dry. Add the yolk to the bread-crumb mixture and fold in the beaten whites. Cook in a small or medium-size, greased frying pan until mixture is set on the top and browned on the bottom. Remove and serve with butter, jelly, or honey. Optional additions are bacon bits and pieces of leftover meat.

Egg Posies

1 hard-boiled egg
1 slice bread, toasted
    and buttered
jelly

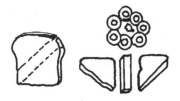

If you happen to have a special tool for slicing hard-boiled eggs into uniform rounds, your three-year-old can probably perform this job for you. If you don't have this gadget, use a serrated knife to slice the eggs (the short way) into 1/4-inch slices. Arrange the slices at the top of a medium-size plate so they overlap and form a flower. Add a dab of jelly in the center. To make the leaves and stem, cut the slice of buttered toast into two triangles and one long strip. Arrange as shown. Voilà!

Hint: If you have trouble with hard-boiled eggs cracking and whites coming out while cooking, try this method. Place eggs in deep kettle. Add cold water to one inch higher than the tops of the eggs. Heat to simmering (190°). Cover pan, remove from the burner, and let set in the hot water for 20–25 minutes (depending on egg size). Run cold water over eggs as usual and peel.

Humpty Dumpty's Reprieve

Scrambled eggs are generally acceptable to the under-five generation. Here are a few suggestions to add a little spice and variety to this old favorite. Add:

- A sprinkling of wheat germ
- Crisp bacon bits, artificial bacon bits, leftover meats or cooked vegetables
- Cottage cheese or any grated cheese
- Drained canned corn (sauté corn in fat and then add eggs)
- Sautéed onion, celery, and/or green pepper
- Seasoned salad croutons

And of course, don't forget **Green Eggs and Ham** (thank you, Dr. Seuss!). You only need **one or two drops of blue or green food coloring** to turn scrambled eggs green. Or try the hard-boiled variation. Crack the shell of an egg but leave it attached to the egg. Place the cracked egg in water with green food coloring for 10 minutes. When the shell is removed, you'll have a green marbled egg.

Breakfast Fruit Combinations

Vitamin C is an important part of breakfast, but again it need not always be served in the traditional orange juice. Consider some of these combinations:

- Apricots and cottage cheese
- Cantaloupe slices
- Grapes, apples, and other fruit with cheese chunks
- Mandarin oranges with sour cream or yogurt
- Orange slices cut into circles
- Sliced peaches and blueberries
- Strawberries and pineapple chunks

When serving an orange, roll it on the counter prior to cutting it to get more juice.

Orange juice is best when freshly squeezed, but frozen is cheaper. Make sure orange-juice cans say "juice"—not "drink"—and also "no sugar added."

From the Griddle

Pancakes and waffles are lots of fun for the whole family. There are prepared mixes for both, plus frozen waffles, which are real time-savers. If you do have the time, here are some basic recipes that just could become a traditional part of your weekend breakfasts.

Buttermilk Beauties

1 cup flour (white, whole
  wheat, or a combination)
1 teaspoon baking powder
1/2 teaspoon baking soda
1 tablespoon shortening
  (melted) or oil

1 egg
1 cup buttermilk (or plain
  yogurt, plus sweet milk
  or water, to make 1 cup
  liquid)

Mix dry ingredients. Add milk and shortening to egg and mix. Combine the two mixtures until they are just moistened. Bake on a hot griddle, browning both sides.

Great Groovy Griddle Cakes

1-1/2 cups flour (white,
  whole wheat, or a
  combination)
1-3/4 teaspoons baking
  powder
3 tablespoons sugar
  or honey

2 eggs
3 tablespoons shortening
  (melted) or vegetable oil
1 or 1-1/4 cups milk

Combine dry ingredients in a large bowl. Beat eggs; add sugar, shortening, and milk. Add wet ingredients to the dry ingredients and mix until barely moistened. Ignore the lumps. Set covered mixture in a cool, dry place for as long as possible (even overnight). Bake on a lightly greased griddle or frying pan. When bubbles appear on upper surface of the cakes, turn and brown on second side.

Cottage-Cheese Pancakes

3 eggs
1 cup cottage cheese
2 tablespoons salad oil or
  butter (melted)

2 tablespoons flour or
  cornmeal

With a small mixer (or a blender) beat eggs. Add cottage cheese and mix until fairly smooth. Add shortening and flour. Make cakes on the "smallish" side. Bake as usual for pancakes.

Personalized Pancakes

Children starting to learn letters and numbers are thrilled to have a stack of pancakes with their initials or age on top of each cake. Offer this on birthday mornings or to celebrate a newly learned letter or number. Here's how you do it!

Dip a teaspoon into pancake batter and let excess drip off. With remaining batter, draw the letter or number *backwards* on the hot, greased pan or griddle. (You might need to practice your mirror-writing on paper first!)

When the underside is lightly browned, pour a spoonful of regular batter over the letter or number so that the pancake will completely surround it. Bake until bubbles appear; then turn and brown second side. The letter or number will appear darker on the finished pancake.

Or try Animal Pancakes, like this:

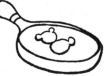

Crumpets

"Tea and crumpets" is an expression that crops up fairly regularly in English novels and films. This recipe creates one of many varieties.

3 cups flour (white, whole wheat, or a combination)
1 tablespoon baking powder
2 tablespoons sugar or honey

2 tablespoons butter or margarine
1 egg
1/2 to 1-3/4 cups milk

Mix flour, baking powder, and sugar. Cut in shortening until mixture is like bread crumbs. Beat egg with milk. Combine wet and dry ingredients and stir just enough to moisten. (The batter should be thick, but if it doesn't spread when dropped on griddle, add some more milk.) Drop batter by tablespoons onto hot, greased griddle. Bake as usual for pancakes.

Thin any leftover batter with a bit more milk to make larger cakes. Use instead of bread for a sandwich.

Wonderful Waffles

2 cups flour (white, whole
   wheat, or a combination)
2 teaspoons baking powder
2 tablespoons sugar or
   honey

2 eggs, separated
2 cups milk
4 to 6 tablespoons
   shortening (melted) or oil

Sift dry ingredients twice. (If using whole-wheat flour, add back particles that didn't go through.) Beat egg yolks, then mix with shortening and honey (if you're using it) and milk. Mix dry and liquid ingredients just enough to blend them. Beat egg whites until stiff and fold into batter. Bake according to manufacturer's instructions for your waffle iron.

Make additional waffles from your leftover batter and freeze them for later use. All you need to do is pop them in a toaster prior to eating. Or if you're super-organized, make the whole batch ahead and freeze them for a series of yummy, fast breakfasts.

Variations on the pancake and waffle theme. To the batter add:

- Fresh or frozen drained berries and a little extra sweetening. (If possible, let batter sit 1/2 hour when adding fresh berries.)

- Chopped nut meats (again, let sit 1/2 hour, if possible).

- Grated orange rind.

- Finely diced ham or bacon bits.

- Nonfat dry milk.

- Or replace part of the flour called for with soy flour, wheat germ, brewer's yeast, or corn meal for more nutritional value.

- Divide batter and add a few drops of food coloring to each batch, so you can offer a colored collection on a platter.

- For waffles—pour batter and then place a piece of uncooked bacon on batter in each section of the iron. Close iron and bake as usual.

Suggested toppings for pancakes and waffles:

- Cinnamon mixed with sugar or honey
- Peanut butter and jelly or honey
- Ice cream topped with wheat germ
- Sweetened apple sauce mixed with sour cream or yogurt
- Canned or fresh fruits, such as peaches, berries, or bananas (roll pancakes around any of the above fruits, secure with a toothpick, and serve the "logs" with syrup and butter)
- The traditional maple syrup or honey and butter

French Toast

French toast is a good way to combine eggs, milk, and bread. If you are going to use homemade whole-grain bread for this purpose, be very careful as you lift the bread slices from the egg-milk mixture into the pan. They are usually more fragile than white bread after being soaked and can break easily.

Here are two batter recipes:

1 egg
1/3 cup milk
1/8 teaspoon vanilla

Or:

1 egg
4 teaspoons flour
1/3 cup milk

For both recipes, beat egg lightly and add next two ingredients. Dip bread into the mixture. Fry in a well-greased pan over fairly high heat, browning well on both sides. Or, on a cold morning, preheat the oven to 500° and bake the dipped bread on a greased pan, turning after the tops brown. Makes approximately 3 slices each.

Serve with any of the suggested toppings for pancakes and waffles.

French-Toast Waffles

1 egg, beaten
1/4 cup milk
2 tablespoons shortening
    (melted) or salad oil

1/2 teaspoon cinnamon
bread slices
1 to 2 tablespoons sugar or
    honey (optional)

Combine all ingredients, except the bread, and mix well. Cut the bread to fit the waffle iron. Dip bread into the batter and bake on a hot, greased iron until well browned. (It may be necessary to hold the top of the iron down for a little while, since the bread has more height than batter alone.)

French Pancakes

1 slice bread (preferably
    whole wheat)
1 egg

1/4 teaspoon vanilla or
    maple extract
1 tablespoon milk

Combine the above ingredients in a blender. Whir until smooth. Cook as for pancakes.

Cereals

Cereal is one of the first foods we give our children, and it generally continues in their diet as a breakfast staple. Historically, cereal began as a nourishing, whole-grain, breakfast food. Processing has changed its food value, but not the tradition. Much has been published about the lack of nutritional value in highly processed dry cereals on the market. Although a child does get some vitamins and minerals, as the cereal manufacturers state, most of the nutritional value comes from the accompanying serving of milk. Some manufacturers spray their cereals with additional vitamins, giving you virtual vitamin pellets, which are not a good substitute for a whole-grain or unprocessed cereal. If you buy fortified breakfast cereals, you may be paying dearly for a few cents' worth of vitamins. According to the Center for Science in the Public Interest in Washington, D.C., Total, for instance, is the same product as Wheaties, except for the sprayed-on vitamins. Note the difference in the prices of these products. Read your cereal labels!

Also, you will find that many of today's popular cereals are mainly sugar—a poor way to start off the day. It is cheaper and more nutritious to add a teaspoon of sugar or artificial sweetener to an unsweetened cereal. Avoid cereals that are sugar-frosted, honey-coated, or chocolate-flavored.

Some cereals that contain no sugars are: Cream of Wheat (farina), Quaker Oats, Shredded Wheat, Nutri-Grain, Kretschmer Wheat Germ, and Wheatena. The sugar in many of the dry cereals tends to encourage children to expect sweets along with the main part of breakfast as well as with other meals.

Hot Cereal

You'll find many kinds of hot, cooked cereals on the market, such as Malt-O-Meal, Roman Meal, Cream of Wheat, Cream of Rice, Oatmeal (the old-fashioned variety), and others. These can be pepped up to look and taste better in any of the following ways:

- Hide one or two chocolate chips in a bowl of cereal for a bit of adventure.

- Add a heaping teaspoon of creamy peanut butter.

- Add raisins, dates, drained canned fruit, frozen fruit, and especially fresh fruit.

- Use any of the above to create a design on the bowl of cereal, such as a face with raisins for eyes and nose, and peach slices for mouth and ears. Draw a spiral design of jelly, or a lacy design à Jackson Pollack, made by drizzling some molasses from a spoon. Use your imagination!

- Add wheat germ, cooked soy grits, and/or nonfat dry milk.

- Serve with a large spoonful of vanilla ice cream.

Homemade Hot Rice Cereal

Grind several cups of raw brown rice to a fine powder in a blender. Store in a tightly covered container. To prepare:

1/2 cup rice powder
2 cups milk
dash of salt

In a small saucepan, bring milk and salt just to boiling point. Add the rice powder, stirring constantly. Lower heat, cover pan, and simmer for 8–10 minutes. Serve with butter or margarine, honey, molasses, wheat germ, fruit, or whatever your family likes. It has a nutty taste.

Corn-off-the-Cob Hot Cereal

1/4 cup yellow cornmeal
1/4 cup cold water
3/4 cup boiling water

2 teaspoons wheat germ (optional)
1/4 cup nonfat dry milk (optional)

Mix together cornmeal, cold water, and wheat germ (if you're using it). Bring the 3/4-cup water to a boil and add the cornmeal mixture and the dry milk (if you're using it). Stirring constantly, bring to a boil and let boil about 2 minutes. Cool and serve with any of the following: butter, margarine, cottage cheese, sour cream, yogurt, jam, honey, brown sugar, maple syrup, raisins, or chopped dates.

Cold Cereal

One idea for making a nutritious and easy bowl of cereal is to crumble a whole-grain muffin in a bowl. Pour milk over it, add fruit, nuts, or sweetener, and you have an instant breakfast.

A popular natural cold cereal on the shelves these days is granola, which is being marketed under a variety of names. Check the list of ingredients carefully, since most granolas have a high-sugar and high-fat content.

Better yet, try making your own granola. It's easy, cheaper, and the proportions of ingredients can be changed around to fit your family's preference. It can also be ground in a blender and served with milk to babies and young children who would choke on the unground cereal. Another way to soften granola is to let it sit in a bowl of milk overnight in the refrigerator.

Granola

4 cups oatmeal, uncooked	1/3 cup vegetable oil
1-1/2 cups wheat germ (raw or toasted)	1/2 cup honey
1 cup coconut, grated	1 tablespoon vanilla
1/4 cup nonfat dry milk	1/2 cup sesame seeds (optional)
1 to 2 teaspoons cinnamon	1/2 cup raw nuts, seeds, or raisins (optional)
1 tablespoon brown sugar	

In a large bowl, mix dry ingredients. Combine oil, honey, and vanilla in a saucepan and warm. Add these to the dry ingredients and stir until all the particles are coated. (Hand mixing works well here.) Spread this mixture in a long, low pan or rimmed baking sheet that has been greased. Bake at *either* 250° for an hour *or* 300° for half an hour, depending on your schedule. (Or **microwave** in a low glass pan 10–15 minutes on high, stirring mixture approximately every five minutes.) Turn with a spatula from time to time. When finished toasting, add dried fruits, such as raisins. Cool and store in an airtight container.

Wheat Germ

Raw wheat germ has greater nutritional value than the toasted kind but is less palatable. So it is probably preferable to use the toasted kind as a breakfast cereal and be assured your kids will like it. Several brands are available, some with additions such as honey and cinnamon. Serve any of these as regular cereal with milk without making a big to-do about it and see what reaction your kids have. Or, if you use raw wheat germ in your cooking and want to toast your own, here's one way to do it:

4 cups raw wheat germ (always keep in refrigerator)
1/2 cup honey, approximately (warmed a bit)

Mix thoroughly and spread mixture on a well-greased baking sheet. Bake at 300° for 10 minutes in bottom third of oven. Cool and store in airtight container in refrigerator.

Additional serving ideas:

- Sprinkle onto peanut-butter sandwiches.
- Mix with other sandwich fillings.
- Add to meat loaf (approximately 1/4 cup).
- Toss a little in a green salad.

Rice Pudding

Usually eaten as a hearty dessert, rice pudding is a nice change-of-pace for breakfast that nonetheless includes milk, eggs, and a grain.

2 cups cooked rice
   (preferably brown rice)
2 cups milk
1/2 cup nonfat dry milk
1/4 cup brown sugar
1 tablespoon butter or
   margarine, melted

2 eggs, well-beaten
1/2 lemon rind, grated
1/2 teaspoon vanilla
1/4 cup raisins
bread crumbs or
   wheat germ

Mix all ingredients together, except crumbs or wheat germ. Grease a 1-quart casserole dish (or individual custard cups) and sprinkle bottom with some crumbs or wheat germ. Pour in pudding mixture and sprinkle more crumbs on top. Bake at 350° for 20 minutes or until a knife inserted in the center comes out clean. (For children, this is best prepared in advance and served cold.)

Breakfast Cookies

Although you may not want to make a regular practice of it, nutritious cookies can be a fun and interesting breakfast as well as a good snack or dessert. Many cookie recipes can be thinned with a little milk and baked in a square pan to make bars, so you have two versions of the same recipe.

Bacon-'n'-Egg Cookies

1-1/4 cup flour (white or whole wheat)
2/3 cup brown sugar
1/2 cup Grape-Nuts cereal
1/2 pound bacon, cooked crisp, and crumbled (or 1/2 cup artificial bacon bits)

1/2 cup shortening, melted
1 egg, beaten
2 tablespoons frozen orange-juice concentrate, undiluted
1 tablespoon orange peel, grated

Mix flour, sugar, Grape-Nuts, and bacon. Add remaining ingredients and blend well. Drop by tablespoonfuls onto a greased cookie sheet (ungreased if you use real bacon) and bake at 350° for 10–12 minutes or until cookies are light brown.

Banana Oatmeal Cookies

3/4 cup shortening
1 cup brown sugar
1 egg, beaten
1-1/2 cups flour (white, whole wheat, or a combination)
1/2 teaspoon baking soda
1 teaspoon cinnamon

1/4 teaspoon nutmeg
1 cup mashed banana
1-3/4 cups oatmeal, uncooked
optional: raisins, nuts, wheat germ, sunflower seeds, grated orange peel

Cream shortening with sugar, add the egg, and mix well. Mix flour, baking soda, cinnamon, and nutmeg together and add to creamed mixture. Blend until smooth. Add mashed banana and oatmeal next. Blend. Drop by teaspoonfuls onto a greased cookie sheet and bake at 400° for 12–15 minutes.

Oatmeal Overnight Cookies

4 cups oatmeal, uncooked
2 cups brown sugar
1 cup bland oil
2 eggs, beaten

1 teaspoon flavoring (vanilla
   or almond)
1/4 cup wheat germ
   (optional)

In the evening, combine oatmeal, brown sugar, and oil. The next morning, add eggs, flavoring, and wheat germ (if desired). Mix well. Drop by spoonfuls onto a greased cookie sheet and bake at 300° for 12–15 minutes. Watch cookies carefully. Remove from sheet while still warm or you may never get them off!

Granola Breakfast Bars

2 cups granola
2 eggs, beaten
dash of vanilla (optional)

Combine the granola and eggs in a greased 8-inch-square pan. Bake at 350° for 15 minutes. Cut into 8 bars. When serving, spread with jam, honey, or peanut butter.

Cereal Balls

1 cup ground-in-a-blender
   cereal (such as shredded
   wheat, granola, or
   wheat germ)

1 tablespoon honey
milk (as much as needed)
1 tablespoon peanut butter
   (optional)

After grinding cereal, add honey and peanut butter. Blend. Add milk until mixture can be rolled into balls. Refrigerate in a covered container.

Variations:

- Roll into logs; roll logs in coconut or wheat germ.

- Add nonfat dry milk and brown sugar, and eliminate peanut butter, liquid milk, and honey. Store in a plastic bag for a convenient treat when traveling. Just add water as needed for a breakfast food or snack.

Creamy Balls

Combine **chopped nuts** and **cream cheese**. Roll into balls and serve.

Quick Breads

If the quick breads in your repertoire of family favorites call for white flour, try substituting whole-wheat flour. Or use the Cornell Triple-Rich Formula (see page 73) with the flour you're using. When substituting whole-grain flour for white, use more baking powder, since whole grains require a bit more help in rising.

Breakfast Banana-Nut Bread

1/4 cup butter or margarine
1/2 cup brown sugar
1 egg, beaten
1 cup bran cereal or
   oatmeal, uncooked
4 to 5 ripe bananas (about
   1-1/2 cups), mashed

1 teaspoon vanilla
1-1/2 cups flour (white,
   whole wheat, or a
   combination)
2 teaspoons baking powder
1/2 teaspoon baking soda
1/2 cup nuts, chopped

Cream shortening and sugar until light. Add egg and mix well. Stir in cereal, bananas, and vanilla. Combine the remaining ingredients in a bowl and add to the first mixture, stirring just long enough to moisten the flour. Grease and flour a loaf pan; pour in batter. Bake at 350° for 1 hour or until bread tests done.

Hint: What to do with that leftover, ripe banana? Mash it, add a bit of lemon juice or Fruit Fresh, and freeze until you make banana bread. If chopped nuts aren't yet appropriate for your child, whirl them in a blender before adding to batter.

Peanut-Butter Bread

2 cups flour (white, whole
   wheat, or a combination)
4 teaspoons baking powder

1/4 cup sugar or honey
1-1/4 cups milk
2/3 cup peanut butter

Lightly mix dry ingredients in a large bowl. If using honey, cream it with the peanut butter in a separate bowl. Heat the milk until lukewarm, then add the peanut butter and blend well. Add the wet and dry ingredients and beat thoroughly.

Pour into a greased loaf pan and bake at 350° for 45–50 minutes. When the bread is cold, make thin slices and spread with honey or jam. This slices best if baked a day in advance and refrigerated after cooking.

Ready Bran Muffins

2 cups boiling water
6 cups 100-percent bran cereal
1 cup shortening (butter, Crisco, or margarine)
2 cups sugar or 1-2/3 cups honey
4 eggs, beaten
1 quart buttermilk

5 cups flour (white, whole wheat, or a combination)
5 teaspoons baking soda
optional additions:
    blueberries, raisins, coconut, peanuts, chopped fresh apples, chopped dates, nuts, a cube of cheese

Preheat oven to 375°. Pour boiling water over 2 cups of the cereal and set aside. Cream shortening with sugar or honey and add the eggs, buttermilk, and the moistened bran cereal, and mix. Fold in the remaining dry ingredients. Fill greased muffin tins 3/4-full and bake 20–25 minutes. Or fill a loaf pan 1/2-full and bake at 350° until done. Batter can be stored in quart jars in the refrigerator for up to six weeks.

Hint: The proportions called for in this recipe make several quarts of batter. If it's too much, cut the recipe in half, give some to a neighbor, or store in the freezer.

Whole-Wheat Muffins

1 cup whole-wheat flour
3/4 cup white flour
1/4 cup sugar or honey
4 teaspoons baking powder

1 egg
1 cup milk
1/4 cup salad oil

Mix dry ingredients. In a separate bowl, beat egg slightly and stir in milk and oil. Add wet ingredients to dry ingredients and stir until just moistened. Batter will be lumpy. Fill greased muffin tins 2/3-full and bake at 400° for 20–25 minutes. Remove muffins from tins immediately after baking.

Orange Muffins

1 slice bread (preferably
   whole grain)
1 egg
1/3 cup nonfat dry milk

1/2 teaspoon baking soda
1 orange, peeled and cut up
1 tablespoon water
4 teaspoons honey or sugar

Put the bread in a bowl and pull apart with a fork. Mix remaining ingredients together and combine with the bread. Spoon into greased muffin cups until 2/3-full and bake at 350° for 30 minutes.

Quickie Turnovers

1 can (8 ounce) refrigerated
   crescent rolls

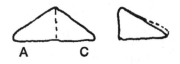

Filling:
1/2 cup honey
1 tablespoon sunflower
   seeds

1 tablespoon raisins
1/4 cup blueberries

Combine all the filling ingredients. Unroll the crescent rolls and place a spoonful of the filling mixture in the middle of each triangle of dough. Moisten the edges of the dough. Following the diagram on the package, fold point A over to point C. Press edges firmly together. Place on a greased cookie sheet and bake at 375° for 10–12 minutes.

Filling variations:

peanut butter
jelly

nonfat dry milk
raisins

   Or:

honey
granola
apple slices

cinnamon and nuts
bread

Bread

The art of baking bread is coming back into its own in this country. If you've never tried it, why not start now? The aroma of yeast bread baking is a delight, one to which you and your family could take a real liking. Being home with small children gives you the type of time slots needed for making bread: five to ten minutes of concentrated work, spread over several hours.

Batter breads are somewhat simpler than breads that must be kneaded, so try a batter recipe if you are a new bread baker.

If baking bread just isn't "your thing," consider using frozen bread dough from your grocer's freezer section. You merely let it thaw and rise, then bake. Most frozen doughs don't contain all those extra ingredients that make bread shelf-stable, but the bread tastes and smells so good that it disappears very quickly. The major disadvantage of this bread is that it is difficult to slice into thin pieces.

You have probably noticed in this book that when flour is called for, the recipe generally gives you a choice of white, whole wheat, or a mixture of the two. Here is what the authors of *The Joy of Cooking* have to say about bleached, enriched white flour:

"After the removal of the outer coats and germ, our flours may be enriched, but the term is misleading. Enriched flours contain only four of the many ingredients known to have been removed from it in the milling."

You can give additional food value to white flour for cakes, cookies, muffins, and breads by using the simple method below, called the Cornell Triple-Rich Formula.

Cornell Triple-Rich Formula

1 tablespoon soy flour
1 tablespoon nonfat dry milk
1 teaspoon raw wheat germ

Place these ingredients in the bottom of your measuring cup before adding flour. Then add flour to make one cup. Do this for each cup of flour you use. Eventually you may want to add a little more of each enricher. Whole-grain flours also benefit from this formula.

Bread-Making Procedures

In case you're wondering how to tell if the bread dough or batter has doubled in bulk, here's an easy way to find out. Press lightly with one or two fingers near the edge of the dough. If a small indentation remains, it has doubled. If not, the dough will spring back.

When bread is browning too fast (turning a light brown after only 10–15 minutes), cover the top lightly with a piece of aluminum foil.

If you've never kneaded, don't let that stop you. You'll improve with practice, so start experimenting now. Kneading is a process of folding the dough and pressing it down with the heel of your hand, over and over again, until the dough is smooth and elastic, not sticky. You may need to sprinkle flour on the dough and your working surface when you begin until the dough loses some of its stickiness.

If you need a warm place, where busy little fingers can't reach, to let your bread rise, place a baking pan filled with about an inch of hot water on the bottom of your oven. Put the bowl or pans of dough that are rising on the middle shelf. You may have to replace water every half hour or so with more warm water. And don't forget to remove the pan of water when you bake your bread!

Or heat your oven to 200° for 60 seconds. Turn off. Then put in bread for rising.

Basic Whole-Wheat Bread

1 cup warm water (105°-115°)	1/3 cup honey
2 packages yeast	1-1/2 tablespoons salt
1 tablespoon honey	5 cups whole-wheat flour
2 cups milk	3 cups white flour
1/4 cup butter, margarine, or oil	1/4 cup wheat germ (optional)

Dissolve yeast in warm water. Stir in 1 tablespoon honey. Set aside for 10 minutes. In a saucepan, combine milk, butter (or margarine or oil), honey, and salt. Heat to lukewarm—do not scald. Pour warm milk mixture and dissolved yeast into a large mixing bowl. Add the whole-wheat flour, one cup at a time, beating well after each addition. Be sure to use all the whole-wheat flour. Add wheat germ, if desired.

Add enough white flour to make a soft, yet manageable, dough. Turn out on a lightly floured board and knead until smooth and elastic, approximately 8–10 minutes.

Place dough in a greased bowl, turning it to grease the top. Cover and let rise in a warm, draft-free place until dough has doubled in bulk. Punch down, divide in half, and knead each half for about 30 seconds.

Shape into three loaves and place in greased loaf pans. Cover and let rise again until doubled in bulk, about 45 minutes.

Preheat oven to 400° and bake 40 minutes or until done.

Cinnamon Swirl Bread

Follow the above dough recipe, but before shaping the dough, roll into three rectangles, about 6" x 16" each. Mix together **4 tablespoons brown sugar** and **4 tablespoons cinnamon;** sprinkle 1/4 cup of this mixture over each rectangle. Beginning with the narrow side, roll up tightly into a loaf; seal ends and bottom by pinching dough together to make a seam. Place in the loaf pans and proceed as in the above recipe.

Refrigerator 100 Percent Whole-Wheat Bread

5 cups milk or water
2 packages dry yeast,
   dissolved in 1 cup warm
   water (105°-115°)
1/2 cup shortening (melted)
   or oil
1/4 cup molasses

1/4 cup honey
11 to 12 cups whole-wheat
   flour (or a combination of
   9 to 10 cups whole-wheat
   and 1 to 2 cups soy flour)
2 tablespoons salt

This recipe is an especially good one if you have an outside job or are too busy during the day with the kids to make bread. Mix the dough in the evening, set it in the refrigerator, and let it rise and bake the next evening. If the dough is to be refrigerated for only three hours, use lukewarm liquid; if it is to be left longer, cool liquid so dough will not rise too much. Dough may still require punching down a few times while it is in the refrigerator.

In a 6-quart pan or bowl, mix together the liquid, dissolved yeast, shortening, honey, molasses, and salt. Add flour gradually, mixing well after each addition. (If using soy flour, add after at least 4 cups of whole-wheat flour have been added.) This dough will be more moist than ordinary bread dough. Let dough rest in the bowl 10–15 minutes.

Turn dough out on a floured board and knead for about 10 minutes, adding as little extra flour as possible. Replace in the bowl, cover with foil or a dampened cloth, and refrigerate immediately for 3–24 hours. Remove from the refrigerator, punch down, and let stand 30–60 minutes at room temperature.

Divide into four equal portions, shape into loaves, and place in four well-greased loaf pans (see hint, below). Lightly grease the tops of the loaves. Let rise in a warm, draft-free place until almost doubled in bulk. Preheat oven to 425°, place pans in oven, reduce heat to 325°, and bake for 1 hour or until done.

Note: This dough makes excellent hamburger buns. Use 1/4 to 1/3 cup of dough for each bun. Bake at 325° for 25–30 minutes or until done.

Hint: If your oven won't hold four pans at one time or you don't own four pans, remove only enough dough from the refrigerator as you can bake at one time. But be sure to take the rest out and use it within 24 hours.

Swiss-Cheese Bread

This bread tastes very nearly like a grilled Swiss-cheese sandwich when toasted. And its braided, glazed top makes it very pretty!

1-1/2 cups milk
2 tablespoons sugar or
 honey
1 tablespoon salt
2 tablespoons butter,
 margarine, or oil
2 cups grated Swiss
 cheese (8 ounces)

2 packages dry yeast
1/2 cup warm water
 (105°-115°)
5 cups white flour
 (approximately)
1 egg and poppy or
 sesame seeds (optional)

Preheat oven to 350°. Scald milk and combine with sugar or honey, salt, shortening, and cheese in a large bowl. (Cheese will probably melt into a lump, but don't worry.) Let cool until lukewarm. Dissolve yeast in the warm water and add to the cooled milk mixture. Stir well. Gradually add flour, stirring well after each addition until a fairly stiff dough is formed.

Knead dough about 5–8 minutes. Place in a greased bowl, turning to grease top; let it rise in a warm, draft-free place until doubled in bulk.

Punch down and divide the dough into two equal portions. Roll each piece out into an 11" x 15" rectangle. Cut each rectangle into three equal strips (the long way), leaving the strips joined at one end.

Braid the strips loosely. Pinch the three ends together. Place each braided loaf in a well-greased pan. Cover and let rise until doubled. Bake 40–45 minutes.

Variation: Just before popping loaves in the oven, beat an egg with 1 tablespoon cool water and brush on tops of loaves. Sprinkle on seeds.

Triple-Rich-Batter White Bread

A good choice for a new baker.

1 cup milk
3 tablespoons sugar or
  honey
1 tablespoon salt
2 tablespoons oil or
  shortening, melted

1 cup warm water
  (105°–115°)
2 packages dry yeast
4-1/4 cups white flour,
  unsifted
Cornell Triple-Rich Formula
  (see page 73)

Scald milk; stir in sugar or honey, salt, and shortening. Set aside to cool until lukewarm (105°–115°).

Add yeast to the warm water in a large bowl and stir until dissolved. Pour warm milk mixture into the yeast. Stir in the flour, one cup at a time, placing the Cornell Formula soy flour, dry milk, and wheat germ in the bottom of the measuring cup first. Beat with a long-handled spoon for about 2 minutes, or longer if using whole-wheat flour.

Cover with a cloth and let rise in a warm, draft-free place until more than doubled in bulk (about 40 minutes). Stir batter down and beat vigorously for about 30 seconds.

Grease two loaf pans, 9" x 5" x 3". Divide batter evenly between them. Batter does not need to rise again. Preheat oven to 375° and bake for about 50 minutes.

Variations:

- Try using part or all whole-wheat flour. Beat a minute or two longer than for white flour.

- Add one or more beaten eggs for a different texture.

Raisin-'n'-Egg Batter Bread

This bread has a rich, cake-like quality.

1 cup milk
1/2 cup sugar or honey
1 teaspoon salt
1/4 cup shortening or
vegetable oil
1/2 cup warm water
(105°–115°)

2 packages dry yeast
1 egg, beaten
4-1/2 cups white flour
1 cup raisins
Cornell Triple-Rich
Formula (optional—see
page 73)

Preheat oven to 350°. Scald milk. Stir in sugar or honey, salt, and shortening. Let cool to lukewarm (105°–115°).

Add yeast to warm water in a large bowl and stir until dissolved. Pour the warm milk mixture into the yeast. Add the egg, and then mix in 3 cups of the flour, beating well after each addition. After the third cup, beat until smooth. Stir in remaining flour to make a stiff batter.

Cover with a cloth and let rise in a warm, draft-free place until doubled in bulk (about 1 hour). Stir batter down and beat in raisins, distributing them as evenly as possible.

Grease two 1-quart casserole dishes or 2 loaf pans, and divide the batter evenly between them. Batter does not need to rise again. Bake for 40–45 minutes or until done.

English Muffins

1 cup milk, scalded
2 tablespoons sugar or
honey
1/4 cup butter, oil, or
margarine
1 tablespoon salt
1 cup warm water
(105°–115°)

1 package dry yeast
5 to 6 cups flour (white,
whole wheat, or a
combination)
cornmeal

This is a good summer bread because you don't have to turn on the oven.

Place hot milk in a large bowl and add sugar or honey, shortening, and salt. Let cool to lukewarm.

Dissolve yeast in the warm water and add to the cooled milk. Add 3 cups of flour and beat until smooth. Gradually add more flour, beating well after each addition until a soft dough is formed.

Turn out on a lightly floured board and knead until smooth and elastic (8–10 minutes), adding more flour as necessary. Place in a greased bowl, turning to grease the top. Cover and let rise in a warm, draft-free place until doubled in bulk (about 1 hour). Punch down and divide in half.

On a lightly floured board, roll the first half out to about 1/2-inch thick and cut as many circles of dough as you can with a muffin cutter (see the hint, below). Gently remove to a cookie sheet that has been heavily sprinkled with corn meal. Sprinkle tops with corn meal, too.

Push scraps together, roll out, and cut again. Continue until you use all the dough. Cover the muffins with a cloth and let rise until doubled.

To bake, heat a griddle or electric fry pan to moderately hot (about 300°) and grease lightly. Using a large spatula, move as many muffins as will fit (without touching) to the griddle. Bake until bottoms are browned (10–15 minutes). Then turn and bake other side.

To cut, insert tines of fork all the way around and pull apart with your fingers.

Hint: A 7-ounce tuna-type can with both ends removed is a perfect cutter for the muffins. But for fun, try cutting them with large, not-too-detailed cookie cutters. (Some won't keep their shape, some will.)

Bagels

1-1/2 cups warm water
(105°–115°)
1 package dry yeast
1 tablespoon salt
3 tablespoons sugar or
honey

4 to 6 cups flour (white,
whole wheat, or a
combination)
1 egg
poppy or sesame seeds
(optional)

Preheat oven to 375°. In a large bowl, mix warm water with yeast; add salt and sugar (or honey). Cover bowl and let stand 5 minutes. Gradually add the flour until a soft-to-medium (but not stiff) dough is obtained.

Knead on a lightly floured board, 5–10 minutes, until shiny and smooth. Add a little more flour as necessary for kneading. Place in a greased bowl, turning to grease the top. Cover and let rise in a warm, draft-free place until doubled, about 30 minutes. Punch down and knead lightly.

To shape into bagels, roll approximately 1/4 cup dough into a strand about 7-inches long and pinch the ends firmly together. Place bagels fairly close together on a floured board or cookie sheet, cover, and let rise again (about 30 minutes) in a warm place.

In the meantime, bring about 5 inches of water to boil in a fairly large, open kettle. Turn heat down so water is simmering. When bagels have risen, gently lift one at a time and drop into the simmering water. Turn them immediately and simmer for about 2 minutes, until puffy but not disintegrating. Several bagels may be put in the water at one time, but do not crowd the pan. Remove the bagels to a towel-covered area to drain and cool while you are boiling the next batch. Place cooled bagels on greased baking sheet. They can be close together.

Beat the egg briefly with 1 tablespoon of cool water and brush mixture over the tops of the bagels. Sprinkle with poppy or sesame seeds, if desired. Bake for 30–40 minutes.

This procedure may look complicated at first, but once you get the knack, you can turn out a batch in 3 to 3-1/2 hours, from start to finish. Makes 12 to 15 bagels.

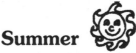

Seasonal Recipes

Here are some seasonal ideas that are often more fun than nutritious, but worth trying on occasion. Many of these recipes yield sugary treats that should be served in moderation.

Summer

Summer means little hands constantly opening the refrigerator in search of things to quench thirst and hunger.

Yogurt Popsicles

1 carton vanilla yogurt
1 can (6 ounce)
   concentrated fruit juice,
   unsweetened (orange
   seems to be a favorite)

dash of vanilla and/or
   honey (optional)

Mix well and freeze in molds (3-ounce paper cups work well). For handles, insert wooden sticks or spoons when mixture is partially frozen.

Variation: Make single servings by mixing some plain yogurt with pureed canned or ripe fruit, or a spoonful of jam or jelly, in a small paper cup. Add a bit of vanilla for extra sweetness, if needed.

Fudgesicles

1 package (4 ounce) regular chocolate pudding mix
3-1/2 cups skim milk
1 egg (optional)

Prepare according to pudding instructions on box. Sweeten to taste. (An egg may be added for extra nutritional value.) Freeze in molds or paper cups and insert Popsicle-stick handles.

Quickie Pops

In a mold or paper cup, mix **apple, pineapple, orange, or grape juice** with **1 teaspoon melted vanilla ice cream.** Mix well and freeze. Add handle when partially frozen. This has the advantage of allowing you to make just one or two rather than a whole batch. Also a good way to get kids to down some orange juice or just use up orange juice left over from breakfast.

Variation: Mash or blend pitted watermelon cubes, pour into a mold, and freeze to make a Popsicle.

Hint: Freeze leftover juices and syrups from canned fruits in ice-cube trays. These add a "perk up" to lemonade or fruit punch. Or insert a stick in the cube before freezing and use as a Popsicle.

Banana Pops

Peel **3 bananas;** cut in half. Push **wooden stick** up center of each half and freeze. Serve this way or dip in **honey** and roll in **toasted wheat germ, nuts, or granola.**

If you have the time and inclination, melt **6 ounces of chocolate chips** (or 12 ounces for 6 bananas) plus a few tablespoons of **water.** Dip the frozen bananas into the chocolate and coat to cover. Twirl to remove excess. After the chocolate sets, wrap in foil and store in the freezer.

Hint: To use up the leftover chocolate, add raisins, nuts, coconut, wheat germ, or what-have-you; drop by teaspoonfuls on a sheet; and cool in the refrigerator for some nutritious candy.

Do-It-Yourself Ice-Cream Sandwiches

Spread **softened ice cream** to the edge of **any appropriate cookie** (graham crackers are good, but most any cookie will do). Gently press another cookie on top. Wrap individually or stack together in foil or plastic wrap and freeze.

Hint: Ice-cream cones are an all-time favorite. Punch a hole in a small foil plate or cupcake paper; place around cone to catch drippings.

Water Ices

Base Syrup:

2 cups water
2 cups sugar

Cook on a low boil for 10 minutes or until approximately at the jelly stage on a candy thermometer. Cool. Use as a base for orange ice, grape ice, or lemon ice, below.

Orange Ice

2 cups fresh orange juice
1/4 cup lemon juice or juice from 1 lemon

Grape Ice

1-1/2 cups grape juice
2/3 cup orange juice
3 tablespoons lemon juice

Lemon Ice

3/4 cup lemon juice
1 tablespoon lemon peel, grated
2 cups water

Pour into trays or a small mixing bowl and freeze. Watch for "mushy" stage (1 hour), then mix in the tray and refreeze. Good alone or served by the scoop in a fruit drink.

Summer Drinks

All drinks seem to disappear from the refrigerator extra-fast at this time of year. The best warm weather drinks are easy to tote and serve. Small juice cans and the disposable boxes of drinks work well. But beverages, like everything else, should be purchased with an eye toward nutrition. Yes, the real juice drinks will cost more. But colored and flavored sugar water is still only sugar water!

Natural fruit-flavored sodas in cans and bottles are popular these days. Though thirst-quenching, these have little nutritional value. Many include only 10 percent fruit juice. For the average, active child, an occasional sugared soda may be preferable. If you do buy sodas, avoid varieties with caffeine, since children tend to be stimulated enough already.

Keeping a good supply of drinks on hand is no easy matter. Here are a few extra ideas:

Apple Juice: Try the frozen or shelf-stable concentrate. It's delicious, sugarless, and economical since it can always be stretched a bit. It can also be reconstituted with sparkling soda for a change of pace.

Flavored Milk: When jam or jelly jars are almost empty, pour in cold milk. Shake and serve as a fruit-flavored drink.

Grape Juice: You can double any amount of grape juice from a bottle by adding an equal amount of water, and for each 2 cups of water added, using 1/2 cup sugar and 1 to 2 fresh lemons. This takes away the "heaviness" from pure grape juice and gives you more for your money.

Fruit Drink: To a glass of lemonade or light carbonated drink add fresh fruit (pineapple, grapes, strawberries, or other favorites) and serve with a fork or toothpick, plus a straw.

Water: Keeping cold water in the refrigerator is an excellent way to encourage consumption of this inexpensive, sugar-free beverage.

Special Touches:

Increase the fun of drinks for a little older child by adding interesting ice cubes. Freeze other fruit juices in ice-cube trays in order to add colors and flavors to those you serve frequently, such as orange juice.

Or make ice cubes more interesting by adding a raspberry, strawberry, or blueberry to ice-cube section before adding water and freezing. They will be noticed in a child's glass.

Topping a drink with whipped cream is always exciting. Add to the interest by sprinkling a few colored sprinkles on the whipped-cream topping.

Lemonade

3 lemons, sliced
1 cup sugar
water

Put lemons and sugar in a 2-quart pitcher or bowl. With a large spoon pound the lemons to release their juice. Stir. Add a batch of ice cubes and let sit awhile, then add water to fill. Mix and serve. Or try:

1 cup reconstituted lemon juice
1-1/2 cups sugar
2 quarts water

Mix and serve.

Summer Picnics

Summer means picnics, whether you camp out or simply cook out. A backyard is as exciting to a child as a national campsite may be to Mom and Dad. And don't forget to use your front stoop for a picnic lunch.

You can simplify any picnic by putting your meal on a skewer! Try a cube of cheese, ham (or any cooked meat), along with pineapple chunks, cherry tomatoes, and pickles on a stick and bagged. Your meal can be eaten right off the stick or slid into a hot-dog bun. The same will work for dessert, whether cookies and marshmallows for toasting or just a selection of fruits.

Finger Jell-O (see page 47) is terrific picnic fare, assuming you're not going to the desert. It does not melt easily.

Don't overlook the magic of a marshmallow roast. Children under three years old will probably eat them uncooked off their stick and still think it's a nifty event. If it's a backyard cookout, let your child invite some neighborhood pals over for a social event of their own.

Take Care

Do not let children run and eat from sticks at the same time. Also beware of sticks with sharp points and sticks from unfamiliar (and possibly poisonous) trees, such as oleander!

S'Mores

large marshmallows
Hershey bars
graham crackers

The traditional recipe! Place a toasted marshmallow and 4 squares of a Hershey bar between 2 graham crackers, and you've done it!

Watermelon Carving

Don't limit your creativity to pumpkins. Make memorable summer shapes from this mouth-watering favorite. In addition to the common "basket" style, how about faces, bunnies, or racing cars?

July 4th—Independence Day

This is the only major summer holiday, so add a little red-white-and-blue to your table.

- Make or buy cupcakes with white frosting and top with several small, red birthday candles. These will simulate firecrackers when lit.

- Use your star cookie cutter to cut out pie dough to create a top star "crust" for a cherry pie.

- Make Finger Jell-O Stars using red-colored and blue-colored Jell-O.

- Use strawberries, blueberries, mini-marshmallows, and Cool Whip, as well as mini-flag toothpicks, to create patriotic dishes and toppings.

- Let your kids ride their bikes and trikes over plastic bubble-wrap for safe fireless "crackers."

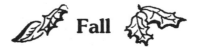 **Fall**

Apple Cider

In a saucepan: Heat apple cider, but do not boil. Add a stick of cinnamon and a few cloves.

In a glass coffee percolator: Put whole spices, such as stick cinnamon and cloves, in the percolator basket. Pour apple juice in the bottom container. Perk a few minutes until cider is spiced to your taste.

Hot-Chocolate Mix

1 box (25 ounce) nonfat
   dry milk
1 jar (6 ounce) Coffee Mate

1 pound instant cocoa
1 cup sugar

Mix well. Store in a covered container. To make as desired, add 3–4 tablespoons mix to 1 cup of boiling water. Stir.

Doughnuts

Use **1 package refrigerated biscuit dough.** Punch a hole in the middle of each biscuit (a bottle cap will work). Fry in **1 inch of hot oil** for about 1 minute or until lightly brown on both sides. Fry the "holes" too. When cool, shake in a bag of **cinnamon** mixed with **sugar, brown sugar, or powdered sugar.**

Popcorn

Children love any and all forms of popcorn *(although popcorn is not recommended for children under three years old).* It's as much fun to make and watch as it is to eat.

TLC Peanut Butter

If you've never made your own peanut butter, now is the time to try a batch. It's a good rainy day (or any day) activity. The challenge is to shell more than you eat!

**1 pound (or less) peanuts in the shell
1 to 2 tablespoons cooking oil
salt (optional)**

Shell, and then chop peanuts in a blender until fine, one cup at a time. Add cooking oil. (Add salt only if peanuts are not salted-in-the-shell variety.) This makes about 1 cup of delicious peanut butter, which should be stored in the refrigerator.

You may also want to experiment with other kinds of nuts, such as almonds, cashews, or walnuts.

The easy way out: Buy peanuts already shelled and toss them in the blender as indicated above.

Spellin' Cookies

**1 package gingerbread mix
1/3 cup water**

With school in progress, help with the homework by making 3-letter cookie words. Combine gingerbread mix with water. Roll out on a floured surface and cut into 3-inch-round cookies. Place them on a greased cookie sheet; with a knife cut the circle in thirds and push the pieces slightly apart. Bake. When cool, make 3-letter words with frosting—a single letter on each piece.

Variation: Use Cuttin' Cookies recipe, below.

Cuttin' Cookies

**3 eggs, beaten
1/2 cup corn oil
1 cup sugar
1 teaspoon vanilla or
   almond flavoring**

**3 cups flour
1 teaspoon baking powder**

Combine all ingredients. Work on a well-floured surface. Roll out and, with cookie cutters or a knife, cut into shapes. (You may wish to chill the dough before rolling out.) Bake at 350° for 8–10 minutes.

Variation:

1/2 cup shortening	1 teaspoon vanilla
1 cup sugar	2 cups flour
1 egg	1 teaspoon baking powder
1 tablespoon milk	1 teaspoon nutmeg

Roll out on a floured surface. Cut into shapes. Bake on a greased cookie sheet at 375° for 6–8 minutes.

Hints:

- Consider using your playdough shape-makers for extra fun and games! Or cut around your child's hand.

- Freeze extra cookie dough in clean frozen-juice cans that are open at both ends. When ready to use, push out, slice, and bake.

Easy Applesauce

several apples	lemon or Fruit Fresh
sweetener	cinnamon
1/4 cup water or apple juice	

Take advantage of the fall harvest by making fresh applesauce. Peel, core, and slice several apples. In a blender place 1/4 cup water or apple juice and add apples one at a time. Blend until smooth. Pour into a saucepan and cook on low heat for 5–10 minutes. Add cinnamon and sweetener (honey or light corn syrup, for example) to taste. A dash of lemon or Fruit Fresh will retard its "darkening" action.

Edible Decorating Glue

Spread **baked cookie** with a thin coating of **honey,** then dip into **shredded coconut, toasted wheat germ, or candy decors.**

Halloween

Halloween is the holiday second only to Christmas in excitement for your child. Full understanding of Halloween comes at a surprisingly early age—costumes and candy, and not necessarily in that order.

Even if you're not planning to make a variety of Halloween food items, don't let that stop you from "renaming" whatever you do prepare on Halloween. Choose from this list for starters:

Bat Bars	Monster Meat (or Munchies)
Devils Delight	Goblin Supreme
Creepy Cookies	Witches Stew (or Brew)
Vampire Vitals	Ghost Gourmet

You can rename peanuts-in-the-shells, "Bats' Knuckles," or bread sticks, "Witches Broomsticks."

To spice up any meal or snack, use your cookie cutter to make a pumpkin face in a piece of cheese or to cut a sandwich into a Halloween shape. Turn Peanut-Butter Balls (see page 49) into spiders by inserting six 2-inch pieces of string licorice. Add just a minidrop of red and yellow food coloring to a glass of milk to turn it into "Pumpkin Punch." Put a gummy worm into a small hole you cut out of an apple for a fun, squeamish snack.

Enjoy carving pumpkins while you can, because by the time your children are in grade school, they will probably take over the responsibility—and the fun. Never carve a pumpkin more than two days before Halloween or it will shrivel up and "die." An ice-cream scoop is a good tool for extracting fiber and seeds. Enhance your jack-o'-lantern by inserting eggshell halves with eyeballs painted on them into the eye holes in the pumpkin.

Use permanent markers to decorate your pumpkins in the weeks before carving, then carve and use them for cooking on or after Halloween. Use a cleaned-out pumpkin for cooking or as a serving bowl. Cookie cutters are good for tracing designs on your pumpkin. You don't have to cut off the top of the pumpkin for a lid; cut a round opening from the bottom instead. To light the pumpkin, simply lower it over a lit candle or a small flashlight.

Roll out peanut-butter balls into small snake shapes and call them crawlers.

Instead of bobbing for apples in water, try bobbing for doughnuts hanging from strings from the top of a doorway. Remember, the trick is still NOT using hands!

Cooked Pumpkin

Use this method to cook pumpkin for a vegetable dish or for pumpkin cake.

Wash pumpkin; cut into large pieces. Remove the seeds and strings or fibers. Put pumpkin pieces, shell side up, in a baking pan and bake in a 325° oven for 1 hour or more, until pumpkin is very tender. (Microwave ovens can do this in less time.) Scrape pulp from the shells; put through a food mill or ricer. If the pumpkin is not thick enough to stand in peaks, simmer it in a saucepan on top of the range for 5–10 minutes, stirring constantly. Freeze in family-size servings.

Toasted Pumpkin Seeds

Don't throw away those wet, string-laden seeds from your pumpkin. They are a delicious treat! Wash the seeds and remove the strings to the best of your ability. Soak the seeds overnight in salted water (1-1/2 teaspoons salt per 2/3 cup water). Then place the seeds in a low baking pan in the oven at 300° for approximately 20 minutes or until golden. Eat with or without removing the shells.

Of course, you can squirrel away a few untoasted seeds and plant them in your garden when spring comes.

Pumpkin Fries

Cut **a small, fresh pumpkin** in half. Peel. Cut into match-stick slices and toss with **2 or 3 tablespoons peanut oil.** Bake on a cookie sheet in a hot oven until brown and tender. Stir often. Sprinkle with **cinnamon** to taste.

Pumpkin Candy

See Fruit Roll recipe on page 52. Use **canned pumpkin** in place of other fruits to tailor this recipe for Halloween.

Pumpkin Cup

Cut a "cap" from an **orange,** preferably the navel variety. Remove the inside pulp and fill with **fruit or candy.** Put a toothpick, which can be used as the eating utensil, on the top of the "cap". Also, scratch a face on the orange and trace the "face" with a ball-point pen so the features stand out, or just use permanent felt-tip markers.

Pumpkin Muffins

1-1/2 cups flour
1/2 cup sugar
2 teaspoons baking powder
1 teaspoon cinnamon
1/2 teaspoon ginger
1/4 teaspoon cloves
1/2 cup raisins
1 egg, slightly beaten

1/2 cup milk
1/2 cup solid pack
    pumpkin, canned
1/4 cup butter or margarine,
    melted
2-1/2 teaspoons sugar,
    mixed with 1/2 teaspoon
    cinnamon

Sift together the first six ingredients into mixing bowl. Stir in raisins. Combine egg, milk, pumpkin, and melted butter. Add wet ingredients to sifted mixture, mixing only until combined. Fill greased muffin pans 2/3-full; sprinkle with cinnamon-sugar. Bake in 400° oven for 20–25 minutes. Makes a dozen muffins.

Hint: Canned pumpkin labels often carry additional recipes and cookbook offers.

Dessert Pumpkins

- To make orange frosting for cakes, cupcakes, or cookies, add equal drops of red and yellow food coloring to white frosting.

- To make black frosting, mix the following together and add to white frosting:

  1-1/2 teaspoons green food coloring
  1-1/2 teaspoons red food coloring
  5 drops blue food coloring

- Candy corn can be used for the eyes, nose, and mouth of a "face."

93

Pumpkin Dessert Cake

See recipe on page 95.

Fanged Favorites

- Cut oranges into quarters and use permanent markers (or carve out spiked teeth) on the rind. Let your little ones sink their teeth into the meat of the orange and show off their new found "fangs."

- Make a terrific "monster mouth" snack by spreading peanut butter on two thin wedges of red-skinned apples to hold together a few mini-marshmallows that look like teeth.

- Turn any pizza into a toothy monster face. Mushrooms, green-pepper slices, cut-up sausage, even candy corn, can top off any cooked pizza into a creative creature.

Hand Horrors

- Fill a disposable, clear plastic glove (not the kind with the interior powder coating) with water and freeze. Dip the frozen glove in warm water and peel off the plastic. Float it in a party punch for a chilling effect.

- Make a fun treat by placing a piece of candy corn in the bottom of each finger of a clear plastic glove (to look like fingernails). Fill the rest of the glove with popcorn or similar treats, tie the wrist closed with a ribbon.

Thanksgiving

This warm, family holiday centers around a large turkey dinner, which most children thoroughly enjoy. It's traditional to stuff a turkey, but try to avoid over-stuffing your children.

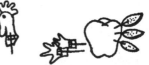

Apple Turkeys

Use an **apple** as the "body." Cut "tail feathers" from **orange peels** and attach with **toothpicks** to the apple. Cut the head and feet from **heavy paper** and **tape** to toothpick "neck" and "legs," which are then stuck into apple.

Candied Cranberries

This holiday snack gives your older toddler a chance to "help."

2 cups fresh cranberries
1 cup water

4 cups sugar
pinch of cream of tartar

Wash berries and dry on a towel. With a small skewer or heavy blunt pin, prick each berry through (or have your toddler do it). Combine 3 cups sugar, 1 cup water, and cream of tartar in a 2- or 3-quart saucepan. Cook over medium heat until mixture reaches 234° on a candy thermometer (soft-ball stage). Remove from heat, pour in cranberries, and stir gently to coat each berry. Let stand at room temperature for at least 12 hours.

Then bring cranberries to a simmer over medium heat, stirring occasionally. Drain berries in a sieve over a bowl. Put syrup back on heat. Bring to a boil and boil rapidly to 250° (hard-ball stage). Remove from heat and dip in cranberries to coat with syrup. Lift berries out with a slotted spoon and cool on wax paper. If a pool of syrup forms around the berry, lift berry to a clean spot. When cool, roll berries a few at a time in the remaining sugar. Leftover syrup can be used on ice cream or for candied fruit.

Pumpkin Dessert Cake

Children are seldom delighted with pumpkin pie. This recipe lets you have your traditional pumpkin dessert, but in a form your children will love.

1-1/4 cup oil
4 teaspoons vanilla
1 cup honey
1 cup molasses or sugar
4 eggs
2 cups pumpkin or 1 can
   (15 ounce) of pumpkin

1/2 cup wheat germ
2 cups whole-wheat flour
1-1/2 cups white flour
2 teaspoons baking soda
2 tablespoons cinnamon
1 tablespoon nutmeg
1 teaspoon ginger

Combine the first six ingredients and mix well. Combine dry ingredients, mix well, then combine with wet ingredients. Mix until blended. Bake at 350° in two greased bread pans for 1 hour or in a 9" x 13" pan for 35 minutes. Top with Cream Cheese Frosting, below.

Variation: You can also make drop cookies from this batter. Bake them at 350° for 10 minutes.

Pumpkin Ice-Cream Pie

1 quart vanilla ice cream
1 can (15 ounce) pumpkin
1/2 cup sugar

prepared pie shell (baked)
  or graham-cracker crust
whipped cream (optional)

Soften ice cream and mix in pumpkin. Add sugar. Freeze in a prepared crust. Top with whipped cream before serving.

Cream-Cheese Frosting

3 ounces cream cheese
6 tablespoons butter or
  margarine

1 teaspoon vanilla
1 tablespoon milk
2 cups powdered sugar

This is a good topping for the Pumpkin Dessert Cake. Mix ingredients and spread on cooled cake or cookies. Extra frosting makes an excellent filler between two graham crackers,

Peanut-Butter Pine Cones

The peanut-butter balls on page 49 can be shaped into small "pine cone" sizes. Using a bag of sliced **almonds** (unblanched), cover the shape with the narrow end of almonds at a 45-degree angle so little of the base shows.

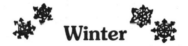

Winter

Take advantage of what is right outside your door—fresh snow! If you find some room in your freezer, pack away clean snow in a plastic bag to use come July, for snow cones, the following recipes, or a mini-snowball fight! *(Not advisable in areas with poor air quality.)*

Snow Mousse

2 cups heavy cream
1-1/2 teaspoons vanilla
1-1/2 cups powdered sugar

large bowl of clean, fresh
  snow

Combine cream, sugar, and vanilla. Whisk in snow gradually, adding more snow until mixture is thick and creamy. Sugar and flavorings may be added.

Easy Ice-Cream Snow

1 cup milk	1/2 cup sugar
1 egg, beaten	1 teaspoon vanilla

Blend the above ingredients well and add clean, fresh snow until mixture is absorbed.

Orange Snow: Spoon some thawed orange-juice concentrate over a dish of snow.

Maple Snow: Pour maple syrup over a cup of snow.

Maple Snow Candy

Fill large pans with fresh, clean, firmly packed snow. Boil real maple syrup until it reaches the soft-ball stage, then pour it in a thin stream from a large spoon onto the snow. After the syrup has started to harden, it can be lifted in sections with a fork and twisted into elaborate shapes.

Christmas Time

Holiday time is an exciting—and often overwhelming—time of the year. It's a wonderful time for cooking up new and old traditions.

Here are some decorating ideas that begin in your kitchen:

- Make cookies to hang on a tree by pushing a plastic straw into a hot cookie just removed from the oven. Twist out a hole at the top. Remove straw. Thread a ribbon through hole.

- String popcorn after it has been allowed to stand long enough to lose its crispness. Popcorn can also be dyed by dipping it in cranberry juice or other colored beverages.

- Or try mini-marshmallows or colored gum drops (cranberries are too hard for small hands to manage).

- To add a cheery note to your table, tie bells on a ribbon around a bread basket.

- Add cinnamon to any playdough you make to add to the holiday fun.

Don't feel you HAVE to bake the Christmas or Hanukkah cookies the kids want to decorate. Buy plain cookies, ready-to-use gels and icing, silver dragies, candied decorations, and colored citrus sliced gummy candies to cut into shapes—and let the kids create-away!

Festive Ideas

- Make "wreath" pancakes and serve with strawberry syrup.

- Serve cooked peas in a scooped-out tomato for its color impact.

- Make a Snack Tree by covering a conical Styrofoam form with green paper. With toothpicks, attach enough edibles, such as cheese cubes, cherry tomatoes, grapes, cauliflower, green pepper, and carrot slices, to cover the tree. Serve with a dip.

- Turn homemade cookies into greeting cards by creating larger ones with personal messages written with tube icing.

- Bake bread in a circle or wreath shape. Press in red and green jelly beans for decorations. Add a ribbon bow after baked bread has cooled.

- Use pointed paper cups for making lime gelatin "trees:" Cut away paper when mold is firm and decorate with cream cheese.

- Create an Orange Sip by rolling an orange between your hands until it is soft. Use a knife to cut an "X" in the orange. Insert a porous peppermint stick in the "X" and sip away!

Christmas Trees à la Rice Krispies

You can devise many holiday treats using the well-known Rice Krispies bar recipe, including these mini-Christmas trees.

5 cups Rice Krispies
1/4 cup margarine or butter
4 cups mini-marshmallows
   or 1 bag (6 to 10 ounce)
   regular marshmallows

10 to 12 regular size
   marshmallows
toothpicks
green food coloring
red cinnamon candies

Melt margarine in a 3-quart saucepan; add 4 cups of marshmallows and cook over low heat. Stir constantly until syrupy. Remove from heat. Add green food coloring until mixture attains a fairly dark green color. Add cereal and stir until well-coated. With buttered hands, shape into conical forms. Cool. Stick a toothpick through a marshmallow and stick into the bottom of the "tree" to serve as the tree base. Decorate with red candies.

Variations:

- **Snowman:** Form three balls of mixture in decreasing size. Roll in coconut, stack, and decorate.

- **Balls:** Shape balls of mixture around a nut or date, then roll in colored sugar.

- **Pops:** Shape pops from the mixture in an oval around a wooden Popsicle stick.

- **Tarts:** Press mixture into a buttered muffin tin to form a tart shell. Fill with fresh fruit or ice cream.

- **Wreaths:** Shape mixture into a "doughnut." Decorate with red candies.

Gingerbread House

1 gingerbread mix
1/3 cup water
Frosting Cement)
   (see page 101)
cardboard
toothpicks

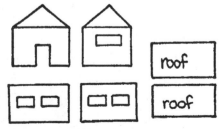

This nifty idea will delight your kids (although not necessarily the nutritionists). Fortunately, it's more to look at than to eat. This simplified recipe does not take a great deal of time.

To one gingerbread mix, add 1/3 cup water. Mix well and roll out into 1/2-inch thickness. It will work best if you take the time to make a cardboard pattern. The base of the house will be about 4" x 6". It will stand about 3-1/2 inches high to the eaves line. You will need 6 sections.

Cut the door and windows before baking, but do not remove the pieces until after baking. Extra dough can be molded into little cookie people. Bake approximately 15 minutes on a greased sheet for maximum hardness, but do not allow the edges to burn. The house is "glued" together with Frosting Cement (see below). Use toothpicks when or where necessary. Use the Frosting Cement to hold the base to the plate so that it will stand. Let the frame dry before adding roof.

If this is more than you want to do, just use frosting cement to attach graham crackers to small milk or orange-juice cartons.

For decoration:

- **Snow Landscape:** Sprinkle coconut around house, or use cotton.

- **Roof:** Spread with icing and cover with mini-marshmallows, coconut, sprinkles, decors, or candied fruit slices, halved. Or use sections of Shredded Wheat to give a thatched-roof effect. Sliced almonds can look like shingles. Add white icing to a few spots to look like snow on the roof.

- **Path:** Build with small circle-candies such as M&Ms, plain chocolate candies, Lifesavers, or sliced gum drops. Build fences with sugar cubes.

- **Chimney:** Pile 2 or 3 hard circle-candies or sugar cubes as a chimney. Cement with frosting.

- **Trees:** Create with green gum drops, lollipops, pine cones, inverted sugar cones, or tree cookies.

- **Snowmen:** Shape 2 balls from leftover frosting. Let dry. Or stack large marshmallows. Attach with frosting.

Frosting Cement

2 egg whites, beaten
1/2 teaspoon cream of tartar
2 cups powdered sugar

A smooth, hard-drying icing. Beat 2 egg whites stiff with 1/2 teaspoon cream of tartar. Add 2 cups powdered sugar and beat 5 minutes with an electric mixer. Since this mixture dries quickly, keep it covered with a damp cloth when not in use.

Traditional Gingerbread Men

2/3 cup butter or margarine
1/2 cup sugar
2 teaspoons ginger
1 teaspoon cinnamon
1/2 teaspoon nutmeg
1 egg

3/4 cup molasses
3 cups all-purpose flour, sifted
1/2 teaspoon baking powder
1 teaspoon baking soda

Put shortening, sugar, spices, and egg in a large mixer bowl. Mix until well blended. Add molasses and mix well. Sift together flour, baking powder, and soda. Stir into shortening mixture and mix well. Refrigerate at least 2 hours for easier handling.

Roll out on floured board and cut gingerbread-men shapes. Use bits of raisin for eyes, nose, and buttons. Sprinkle with granulated sugar, if desired. Bake on greased cookie sheets at 375° for 8–10 minutes. Makes about a dozen 5-inch gingerbread men.

Hanukkah Hints:

- Use Hanukkah cookie cutters on Finger Jell-O (blueberry and lemon flavors) for appropriate symbols of the seasons.

- Use the play-clay recipe on page 115 to form festive menorahs.

- Make decorative holiday placemats by drawing with blue crayons on beige or yellow inexpensive vinyl mats.

- Spray menorahs with nonstick vegetable shortening before lighting candles for quicker cleanup.

Potato Latkes

Let kids help make the traditional Potato Latkes each year. Grate **3 peeled potatoes** and a bit of **onion.** Squeeze out excess liquid and drain. Add **2 beaten eggs** and **2 tablespoons flour.** Fry small dollops of batter in minimal **oil** until brown. Turn and cook until crispy. Drain on paper towels and serve with **sour cream and/or applesauce.**

Valentine's Day

Valentine's Day is a day to make good use of your heart-shaped cookie cutter—on toast, sandwiches, cheese slices, red Finger Jell-O, and, of course, on cookies!

Lollipop Heart Cookies

Use the Cuttin' Cookies recipe on page 89. Roll dough out thinly and use heart-shaped cookie cutters. Place dough hearts on a cookie sheet with extra space between rows. Take flat, wooden Popsicle sticks that you've soaked in cold water for an hour and place half-way down heart, making a 2" handle. Then take another dough heart on top; press edges and shape gently together. After they've cooled, decorate with white icing or frosting with red decors. Or dip in melted semi-sweet chocolate chips (let excess drip back into pan) and cool on wax paper. Add sprinkles or decors before refrigerating to harden.

Valentine Krispies

Use the Rice Krispies marshmallow-bar recipe (see Christmas Trees on page 99). Add red food coloring to the syrup just before mixing it with the dry cereal. Mold in a heart-shaped, greased cookie cutter. Take it out and put on a plate to cool.

Need a heart-shaped cake pan, but have no such pan? Bake a round and a square layer cake (8-inch or 9-inch) and combine them this way:

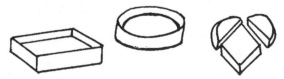

Spring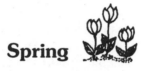

The egg is often used symbolically as part of Easter and Passover celebrations. It symbolizes new life in both traditions.

An Easter egg hunt—indoors or out—is always great fun. Add some hidden peanuts-in-the-shell to provide extra hunting fun. *(Always keep an accurate count of eggs hidden indoors!)*

Decorating Easter Eggs

Use hard-boiled eggs, since they can best take the stress of handling by small children. Take advantage of food coloring in your pantry. Let your eggs soak for at least half-an-hour in bowls of hot water with different colors in each. After removing, let them dry and decorate them with nontoxic magic markers. It's a great medium and easy for kids to handle. An egg carton or a cardboard tube cut into sections makes an excellent drying and decorating stand. When finished, put a drop of shortening on your hands and rub over each egg to give it a shine and to set the color. You can also glue on additions such as ribbon, rick-rack, and even plastic "eyes." Serve decorated hard-boiled eggs throughout the Easter season.

Egg-Shaped Cookies

Make an egg-shaped cookie cutter by bending and shaping the open end of a 6-ounce juice can. Decorate with a variety of icings or with Egg-Yolk Paint (see recipe below).

If you're not up to making your own dough, use a roll of refrigerated sugar cookies and shape.

Egg-Yolk Paint

Blend **1/4 teaspoon water** with **1 egg yolk.** Divide among several small dishes and put different food coloring into each dish. Paint designs on cookies before baking.

103

Jell-O Eggs

Save **egg shells** (either blown-out ones or half shells). Rinse and let stand at least a day. Fill with **Finger Jell-O** (see page 47). Crack and remove shell after Jell-O has hardened. Regular Jell-O can also be used here, but use half of the cold water called for.

Also, you can turn any Finger Jell-O recipe into pastel colors by dissolving **two 4-ounce packages of gelatin** in **1 cup of boiling water.** After it cools to room temperature, whip in **8 ounces of Cool Whip** (in place of additional water) and combine with the 6 ounces of Jell-O dissolved in 1 cup boiling water. After firmed up in the refrigerator, use bunny or egg-shaped cookie cutters to create pastel treats.

Egg Tree

A branch can be decorated attractively using decorated egg shells. Here you must blow out the inside of the raw egg before decorating and hanging it. Use glue to affix strings. If a budded branch is put in a narrow-necked vase with water, leaves will soon adorn the branch along with the decorated eggs.

Bunny Salad

Place a **canned pear half** on a bed of **lettuce.** Add **raisins** for eyes, a **strawberry** (with a toothpick) for the nose, toothpicks for whiskers, and **thin-sliced cheese** (or paper) for the ears.

Bunny Biscuits

Use **refrigerated biscuits.** Cut one in half horizontally, then cut one of those pieces in half to use as the head. Cut the remaining piece in half for the ears. Pinch out a bit for the tail and bake as directed.

Bunny Ice-Cream Dish

Arrange **3 balls of vanilla ice cream** on a plate to form a bunny. Use a large one for the body, a medium one for the head, and a small one for the tail. Cover with **shredded coconut.** Use **jelly beans or almonds** for the eyes and nose, paper cutouts for the ears, and toothpicks or licorice string for whiskers.

Bunny Cakes

Version One: Bake a cake in a heart-shaped pan and cover it with white or pink frosting. Decorate it as shown in the diagram below, using paper cutouts for ears, jelly beans for eyes and nose, and icing or licorice string for whiskers.

Version Two: Bake cake in one-layer cake pan. Cut layer in half, as shown. Stand layers side by side, attaching them with a filling of your choice. Shape rabbit by cutting out notch to make a body and head. Use notch for tail. Frost with fluffy white frosting and sprinkle with coconut. Insert paper ears, jelly beans for eyes and nose, and licorice strings for whiskers. Sprinkle green-tinted coconut and more jelly beans on the cake platter.

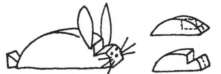

Tinted Coconut: Add a few drops of food coloring to a small amount of water in a bowl; add coconut and toss with a fork until evenly distributed. Or, in a small jar, toss 1-1/2 cups coconut with 1 to 2 tablespoons fruit-flavored Jell-O. Shake well.

Easter Baskets

- Use a pipe cleaner as a handle on a margarine tub. Fill with seedless green grapes.

- Decorate a frosted cupcake with green-tinted coconut. Use pipe cleaners to form basket handle.

- Weave ribbons in and out of green, plastic berry baskets, and add a handle and some plastic "grass" for a quick, colorful basket.

- Turn a third of the bottom part of an egg carton into a decorative egg holder. Paint the section, add a handle (pipe cleaners) with a bow, and kids can easily carry four eggs safely.

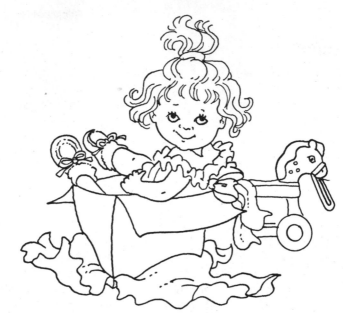

So You're Having a Birthday Party!

Here are a few insights to help you make your child's birthday party the happy time it's supposed to be:

- Plan ahead.

- Keep it short and simple.

- And, above all, keep it moving!

The most important "rule" is one that is often the most difficult to follow:

- **The number of juvenile guests should not exceed the number of years in your child's age.**

Keep in mind that young children enjoy most what they know best. This is not the age for surprise parties. Build on tradition—offer the same songs, cakes, balloons, candles, gifts, and games that have always been favorites.

For more party ideas for these ages, see Vicki Lansky's *Birthday Parties: Best Party Tips and Ideas* (Book Peddlers).

Year One

This party is really for adults. At least one set of grandparents plus an aunt, a cousin, an uncle, the baby-sitter, a neighbor, or friend will want to attend. The food can be fancy and oriented towards adults because your baby will care very little about it, unless he or she can get hands into the goo or the ice cream. Your child will be bewildered by the presents but truly enjoy the attention, excitement, and picture taking.

If the party also includes mothers with their small children, consider a BYOHC (bring your own high chair) party. Provide disposable bibs, travel Baby Wipe packages, and teething biscuits as favors. Have film and your camera ready. There is only one first birthday party!

Limit the party to an hour.

Year Two

By the second year, the miracle of maturation gives your child a clear understanding of a birthday party, its food, and its presents. Keep the party as small—yes, as small—as possible. Two-year-olds are a bit young for games yet. A supply of toys and balloons works well. Since sharing is not usually a strong point at this age, you may spend some time refereeing. Odds are you'll also be entertaining the mommies and possibly the daddies.

A good food idea for the children is something simple, like cupcakes and/or ice-cream cones with sprinkles. Disposable bibs and Baby Wipes may still be in order. The birthday cake with the candles may be for the adults, but only after its candles are blown out and the children are served their share. Don't waste good food on the kids—they usually don't eat more than a few bites.

Limit the party to an hour or an hour and a half.

Year Three

Now you are entering the realm of the more traditional birthday party. Games can be played and enjoyed, although they must definitely be led. Keep it simple. Three to five short games should suffice. Avoid competitive games unless everyone can get a prize. A quiet game or storytelling is a better prelude to refreshments than active games. (See the list of games at the end of this chapter.)

Your three-year-old can begin to learn the social graces. Manners won't be perfect, but this is a good starting point. Greeting guests, opening presents, verbalizing thanks, and saying good-bye are concepts to be discussed before the party and congratulated on afterwards.

Your child should also be consulted about the guest list. He or she can help mail or deliver the invitations and help choose or frost the cake. Written thanks for presents are not necessary.

Food should again be simple. If you are dying to try an unusual form cake, don't. Children do enjoy form cakes; just don't get carried away. Three-year-olds judge most cakes by their icing alone.

Also save yourself time and hassle by scooping out ice-cream balls ahead of time. Place them in a cupcake paper and store in the freezer until you're ready for them. Or buy ice-cream cups and serve them with their wooden spoons.

A fun place card is a cookie with each child's name written on it in icing. Or let each child decorate his or her own cookie. Provide icing, a Popsicle stick, and decorations such as sprinkles, nuts, raisins, chocolate chips, and coconut.

Do include a "hunt" (for candy, peanuts, or other prizes) in your party. A party hat or small plastic bag is an appropriate holder. Save some extra goodies in case any child totally misses the boat.

While candy is an integral part of any party, you may want to include more nutritious treats. Consider these:

chocolate- or yogurt-covered raisins
Finger Jell-O (see page 47)
Fruit Roll (see page 52)
peanuts in shells
pretzels tied with ribbons
raisins, nuts, and sunflower seeds
sugarless bubble gum
Uncandy Bars (see page 50)

A favorite treat that makes a birthday special is Candy Cookies, below. Bake them either for a party at home or at nursery school. If you add the candies to the cookie tops and use the Cornell Triple Rich Formula, you'll compromise the kids' love for candy with a bit of nutrition.

Limit the party to an hour and a half.

Candy Cookies

1 cup oil
1 cup brown sugar, packed
1/2 cup sugar
2 eggs
2 teaspoons vanilla
1-1/2 teaspoons baking
  soda

2-1/4 cups flour
  (see Cornell Triple-Rich
  Formula, page 73)
1 cup (or less) M&Ms Plain
  Chocolate Candies

Cream oil, sugars, eggs, and vanilla. Mix dry ingredients and combine with creamed mixture. Drop by teaspoonfuls on an ungreased cookie sheet. Flatten to not more than 2-inch diameter. Decorate with 4 to 6 candies per cookie, but do make sure (to avoid being hassled) that the number of candies is the same for every cookie.

Bake at 375° for 8–10 minutes. The candies often crack after baking. This recipe makes 2–4 dozen cookies, depending on the size of your teaspoonful.

We can offer no advice on presents, prizes, or party favors. You alone must live with your budget and your neighbors. But remember, *more* does not mean *better.*

Year Four

Most of what goes for a three-year-old's party is applicable here—and more so. By now, the moms and dads are no longer on the sidelines to help, so it's up to you to keep the ball rolling. If it's too much for you to be leader, song director, photographer, server, and clean-up committee, have someone help you—possibly a neighborhood teenager.

Alleviate the awkwardness of the party's start, while you're waiting for all the guests to arrive, by having a planned activity.

String a birthday necklace, decorate a favor bag, or even open the presents.

Four-year-olds anticipate games eagerly. A variety of short games is good for their short attention spans (see the list at end of the chapter). In addition to some games, a clown or puppet show would be a treat. Check on the talents of some of the older children in your neighborhood.

You may find yourself holding the party around lunch or dinner. Here are foods with the best chance of being eaten:

Grilled cheese sandwiches
Pizza
Macaroni and cheese
Hamburgers
Peanut-butter-and-jelly sandwiches (cut with cookie cutter)
Potato chips (individual bags are a treat)
Carrot sticks
Dill pickles
Apple wedges
Mandarin oranges
Green grapes (seedless)
Juice (apple, pineapple, orange)
Chocolate milk

Sandwiches should be "crustless!" After all, this is a party. Avoid drinks that stain. Juice boxes are special as well as spill-proof!

Make portions small. Children often eat very little because they are too excited.

For a different ice-cream treat, cut off the tops of some oranges and scoop out the inside. Put in orange sherbet and freeze until ready to serve.

Consider Do-It-Yourself Sundaes, letting the children help themselves to their favorite ice-cream toppings: fudge, honey, maple syrup, granola, nuts, crushed pineapple, coconut, and whipped cream.

Or make a clown cone. Top a scoop of ice cream with a sugar cone for a hat and decorate a face on it. Reddi-Whip makes good "hair." Make ahead of time and freeze.

Do not feel you have to seat a group of children in your dining room. Any appropriate room with a vinyl tablecloth on the floor and low tables (coffee table, card tables on books, or bricks) will work just fine.

While you can specify a pick-up time, returning your guests to their homes lets you end the party on your schedule.

Limit the party to two hours.

Year Five

While home parties for this age are still recommended, away-from-home parties will now also work for kids. Avoid movies but check out hamburger franchises, pizza parlors, ice-cream parlors, gymnastics programs, skating rinks, and even your local zoo.

Birthday Party Dangers

Beware of:
- Little girls with long hair trying to blow out candles (hair burns).
- Children running with straws or lollipops in their mouths.
- Children playing with (and choking on) uninflated or broken balloons.

Preschool Games

Let your birthday child be the first to be IT in a game.

Plan more games than you think you'll need in case some turn out to be too hard or unpopular. On the other hand, don't feel you must play all the games you planned—or any the birthday child doesn't like or isn't good at.

The younger the guests, the more likely they may not want to play every game, so have alternatives, such as coloring books or puzzles, available.

Games are listed in progressive order for younger children, ages two to three, to older children, ages four to five.

- **Ball roll:** Sitting in a circle with legs spread, children roll a ball from one to another.

- **Tell a story:** Read from a book with large pictures or use your imagination. Keep it short.

- **Action songs:** Ring-around-the-Rosy; Farmer-in-the-Dell; London Bridge; Eensy Weensy Spider; Hokey-Pokey.

- **Animal parade:** March around as an elephant, a bunny, a dog, a cat, a bird, a kangaroo, or another animal.

- **Pin the Tail on the Donkey:** Or "pin" the nose on the clown.

- **Drop (or toss) a bean bag into a basket.**

- **Simple Simon:** Keep it simple!

- **Balloon push:** Outside, it can be done by kicking; inside, by crawling and using one's nose.

- **Kangaroo race:** Hop, holding a balloon between the knees.

- **Ring the bell:** Hang a bell in a tree outside or in a doorway inside; children throw a bean bag or Nerf ball at the bell so it will ring when hit.

- **Musical chairs:** The way you remember it or a variation. Pass a plastic or tin plate; the holder when the music stops is "out."

- **Dress up:** Have a large pile of oversized clothes, hats, and shoes that kids all race to get into simultaneously (take photos).

- **Duck, Duck, Gray Duck:** A circle game of catch.

- **Doggie, Doggie, Who's Got the Bone?:** Children sit in a circle; one in the center is blindfolded and an object is given to another child. Then all children put their hands behind their backs and the group recites, "Doggie, Doggie, where's your bone? Someone has taken it far from home!" With blindfold off, the child now is given three chances to guess who has the "bone."

- **Shoe race:** Everyone removes shoes and places them in a pile. On signal they race to find and put on their own shoes (without buckling, fastening, or tying) and race to the finish line.

- **Bingo!**

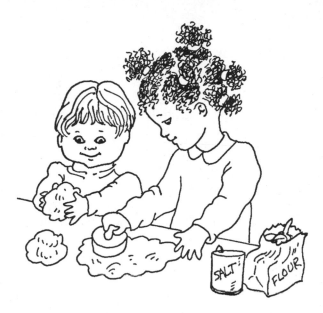

Kitchen Crafts

Work and play are not separate in a child's world—they are inseparable. The same goes for their relation to you—you work and they play! Your time is often spent in the kitchen and your child's will be too, so give your child a chance to do some creative "messing around"!

The first opportunity is the kitchen itself, with all the grown-up tasks to be done. Many of these can be shared with your youngsters. Don't expect perfection; remember they are new to these tasks.

- Washing dishes, dirty or not.

- Setting the table.

- Folding napkins.

- Washing and cleaning vegetables.

- Scrubbing the floor.

- Cleaning your kitchen sink—it will be spotless.

Doughs, Clays, and Pastes

Your kitchen can serve as the starting place for many fun activities. If you've never made your own modeling clay, now is the time to start. Following are three recipes, each with special characteristics. Experiment to find your favorite. (Your child's age may also determine which you'll use.)

When using any form of modeling clay, don't neglect those necessary pieces of equipment: cookie cutters, rolling pins (real or play), plastic knives, bottle caps, extra flour, uncooked spaghetti or macaroni, walnut half-shells, and others, limited only by your and your child's imaginations.

No-Cook Playdough

1 cup white flour
1/2 cup salt
2 tablespoons vegetable oil

1 teaspoon alum
food coloring
1/2 cup water

Mix first four ingredients. Add food coloring to the water. Gradually add small amounts of water until mixture attains the consistency of bread dough. You may not use the entire 1/2 cup of water. You can make colors not commercially available, such as purple, by creatively mixing colors. Store in an airtight container or plastic bag. It lasts a long time. (If you can't find alum at the grocery store, look in the drugstore.)

Stove-Top Playdough

1 cup white flour
1/4 cup salt
2 tablespoons cream of
  tartar

1 cup water
2 teaspoons vegetable food
  coloring
1 tablespoon oil

Mix flour, salt, and cream of tartar in a medium pot. Add water, food coloring, and oil. Cook and stir over medium heat 3–5 minutes. Mixture will look like a globby mess and you'll be sure it's not turning out, but it will. When it forms a ball in the center of the pot, turn out and knead on a lightly floured surface. Store in an air-tight container or plastic bag. Edible but not as tasty as Playdough à la Peanut Butter!, our third recipe!

Playdough à la Peanut Butter

18 ounces peanut butter	nonfat dry milk or milk plus
6 tablespoons honey	flour, to the right
cocoa or carob (optional)	consistency

Mix. After shaping, decorate (try raisins) and eat!

Another edible playdough can be made from one can of frosting, 1-1/2 cups powered sugar, and 1 cup peanut butter.

When your child is old enough to appreciate something a bit more permanent, add "real" homemade clay to your bag of tricks.

Clay for Play and Posterity

Baking Method:

1 cup salt	2 tablespoons vegetable oil
1/2 cup water	2 cups flour

Mix salt, water, and oil. Add flour. After shaping, the clay can be baked at 250° for several hours.

Overnight Drying Method:

1 cup cornstarch	food coloring, tempera, or
2 cups baking soda	acrylic paints (optional)
(1 pound)	shellac or clear nail polish
1-1/4 cups cold water	(optional)

Mix cornstarch, baking soda, and water. Stir in a saucepan over medium heat for about 4 minutes until the mixture thickens to the consistency of moist mashed potatoes. Remove from heat, turn out onto a plate, and cover with a damp cloth until cool. Knead as you would bread dough. Shape as desired or store in airtight container or plastic bag.

To color, add a few drops of food coloring to the water before mixing it with starch and soda. Or, objects may be left to dry, and then painted with tempera or acrylics. Dip in shellac or brush with clear nail polish to seal.

Clay Christmas Ornaments
(Oven Drying Method)

4 cups flour	food coloring, poster paints,
1 cup salt	acrylic paints, or markers
1 teaspoon alum	clear shellac, spray plastic,
1-1/2 cups water	or nail polish

Mix ingredients well in a large bowl. If the dough is too dry, work in another tablespoon of water with your hands. Dough can be colored by dividing it into several parts and kneading a drop or two of food coloring into each part. Roll or mold as desired. (If you can't find alum at the grocery store, look in the drugstore.)

To Roll: Roll dough 1/8-inch thick on lightly floured board. Cut with cookie cutters dipped in flour. Make a hole in the top, 1/4-inch from the edge, with the end of a plastic straw dipped in flour. Shake the dots of clay from the straw and press on as decorations. Thread ribbon or wire through the hole to hang ornament.

To Mold: Shape dough into figures (such as flowers, fruits, and animals) no more than 1/2-inch thick. Insert a fine wire in each for hanging.

Bake ornaments at 250° on an ungreased cookie sheet for about 30 minutes. Turn ornaments over and bake another 1-1/2 hours until hard and dry. Remove and cool. When done, sand lightly with fine sandpaper until smooth. Paint with food coloring, plastic-based poster paint, acrylic paint, or markers. Paint both sides. Allow paint to dry and seal with clear shellac, spray plastic, or clear nail polish.

This recipe makes about 5 dozen, 2-1/2-inch ornaments.

Clay Cookie Ornaments
(Overnight Drying Method)

2 cups salt 　　　　　　　1 cup plus, cornstarch
2/3 cup water 　　　　　　1/2 cup cold water

Mix salt with 2/3 cup water and boil. Add cornstarch and remaining water. Stir. If mixture doesn't thicken, set back on the stove. Sprinkle extra cornstarch on table and rolling pin. Roll out dough and cut with cookie cutters. Use a plastic straw to make hole at the top for hanging. Dry and decorate. Use paint, glitter, and so on to decorate. *These are not edible!*

Bread Clay Recipe

6 slices white bread 　　　1/2 teaspoon detergent or
6 tablespoons white glue 　　2 teaspoons glycerin
1 teaspoon white vinegar 　food coloring

Whoever said that plain, old white bread isn't worth anything! Remove the crusts from the bread and knead bread with white glue, vinegar, and detergent or glycerin. Knead mixture until it becomes nonsticky. Separate into portions and tint with food coloring. Shape and when done, brush with equal parts glue and water for a smooth appearance. Let dry overnight to harden. Acrylic paints, plastic spray, or clear nail polish will seal and preserve your child's art "treasures."

Homemade Silly Putty/GAK-Like Goo

2 parts Elmer's white glue
1 part Sta-Flo Regular liquid starch

Mix well. Putty must dry a bit before it is workable. It may be necessary to add a bit more glue or starch; you will have to experiment. Some suggest equal parts; others have success with starch to glue 2:1. (*Recipe may not work well on a humid day.*) Store in an airtight container. Beware of contact with clothes and carpet. If you use Elmer's school glue instead of regular white glue, it doesn't bounce or pick up pictures, but it makes a gooey delight your kids will love. Use on a smooth surface.

Alternative: Combine 8 ounces of Elmer's white glue and 3/4 cup colored water. Then add a mixture of 1 teaspoon of 20 Mule Team borax and 2 tablespoons of water. Stir until a blob forms and remove from mixture. Continue adding borax mixture until you have enough globs to knead together. Store in airtight container.

You will probably find yourself supporting Borden's Company (makers of Elmer's) by buying both its regular glue and its more washable school glue. But home paste will work for many projects.

No-Cook Paste

a handful of flour
water
a pinch of salt

Gradually add water to flour and mix until gooey. Add salt. This recipe can also be used as a quickie finger paint by adding some food coloring and working it on heavy paper or cardboard. Also works well as a papier-mâché paste.

Library Paste

1 cup flour   4 cups water
1 cup sugar   oil of cloves or wintergreen
1 teaspoon alum

Mix first four ingredients in a saucepan. Cook until clear and thick. Add 30 drops oil of cloves or wintergreen and store in a covered container. (If you can't find alum at the grocery store, look in the drugstore.)

Glass Glue

2 packets unflavored gelatin
2 tablespoons cold water
3 tablespoons skim milk

In a bowl, soften gelatin in cold water. Heat milk to boiling and add to soften gelatin. Stir until gelatin dissolves and pour into a jar.

Use this when something must adhere to glass, such as labels on jars, or to glue wood to wood. Keeps only a day or two. Set jar in a pan of hot water to soften for reuse.

Lightweight Glue

Egg white makes a good adhesive for constructing kites. It is strong and almost weightless. Liquid starch and corn syrup work as glue on many projects, especially for facial decorations at Halloween time. It allows cotton or oatmeal to adhere to kids' faces.

Finger Paints

Finger painting does not occupy the attention of small children for as long as we would wish (cleaning up always seems to take longer than playtime). But it's worth the effort for the discovery and fun value. Do not show your child how to use finger paints as you think they should be used—experimenting is the best part for your child. Sometimes, it is fun for him or her just to feel the cool, smooth paint and see the bright colors. A linoleum floor, covered with newspapers, is often the best painting place since it often has to be cleaned after a painting session anyway! Regarding regular water-based paint: Powdered poster paint is a good investment. It can be found in art-supply or crafts stores and lasts a long time.

#1 Finger Paints

3 tablespoons sugar
1/2 cup cornstarch
2 cups cold water
food coloring
pinch of detergent

Mix the sugar and cornstarch, and then add the water. Cook over low heat, stirring constantly, until well blended. Divide the mixture into four or five portions and add a different food coloring to each, plus a pinch of detergent (to facilitate cleanup).

#2 Finger Paints

1/2 cup dry laundry starch
1/4 cup cold water
1-1/2 cups boiling water
1/2 cup soap flakes
1 teaspoon glycerin
food coloring

Mix starch and cold water in a saucepan. Pour in the boiling water and cook over low heat until shiny. Remove from the heat and add soap and glycerin. Divide the portions and add different food coloring.

Soapy Finger Paints

Beat **warm water** into **Ivory Flakes** to desired consistency and add **paint or food coloring.**

If you don't wish to go to the trouble of mixing finger paints, add **a drop of food coloring** to **aerosol shaving soap** and let your child do his or her thing on a cookie sheet.

Canned Kid Paint

Here's a quickie. Just add **food coloring** to **sweetened condensed milk** that you've divided into different small bowls.

Brushes

- Try a pastry brush if you can spare yours. These have wider handles, and the stiffer brush cuts down on splatters.

- Or try cotton swabs. A different swab can be used for each color so that paint (hopefully) remains unmixed and bright.

Face Paint

Mix one part solid **shortening** (like Crisco) to two parts **cornstarch.** Combine with **food coloring** for desired effects. Add enough **glycerin** to allow the paint to spread smoothly on the skin.

Printing

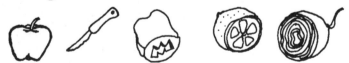

Printing—Vegetable Style

Cut a **potato, carrot,** or **turnip** in half and carve out a raised design (Mom or Dad's job). Brush **poster paints** over the design. Or stamp the design in an **ink pad.** Press firmly on paper: white tissue paper, uncoated shelf paper, ribbons, or anything you have around. Let dry.

Sliced citrus fruits, apples, and even onions also make lovely prints.

Printing Utensils

While sponges, plain or cut into shapes, are the most obvious printing utensils, also try some of the following: a potato masher, wooden salad fork, extract bottle bottoms, and toothbrushes.

Paper Product Paraphernalia

Here are just a few ideas for using everyday items.

Straws

To make any day special, and perhaps to encourage drinking a disliked beverage, try this trick. Make a cut-out (one paper plate will provide several) in a circle or special shape. Use a hole puncher to make a hole in the top and bottom of your design. Decorate or let your child do so, then weave the straw in one hole and out the other. (If you include names on your design, these could be dandy "place cards" for a birthday party.)

Paper Plates

These can be made into clocks, puppets, or hats.

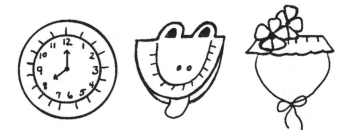

Milk Cartons

There are many things you can do with your empty milk cartons. Consider this fun idea:

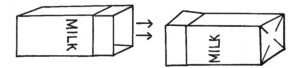

Make building blocks: Use two milk cartons of the same size. Open the top ends completely, then slide cartons together (as shown) to make a block. Cover with Contact paper to decorate.

Paper Cups

These can be made into:

- **Bells:** Decorate.

- **A minidrum:** Cover top with paper and hold in place with an elastic band.

- **A telephone:** Connect two cups with a long string.

- **Spy glasses:** Attach two cups with tape, punch holes for eyes, and use string to secure around the head.

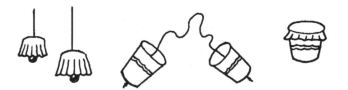

Brown Paper Bags

- Large brown bags make good life-size masks and costumes for young children. Help children cut facial features and holes for their arms and let them do the rest alone.

- Brown bags can also be decorated even when they will later be used as garbage bags.

- To make a flashlight face, cut out features on the base of a bag and insert a flashlight. Twist the bag around the handle and fasten with tape, leaving an opening for the switch.

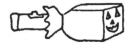

- A smaller bag makes an excellent hand puppet. (Make the "head" on the base of the bag.)

- Or make a tote bag:

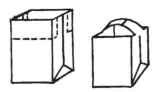

Turn a handled plastic bag into a disposable food or art "bib." Cut across the bottom and up one side between the two handles. Use the handle "holes" for arm holes.

Miscellaneous Fun

Stained-Glass Crayons

A good way to use all those broken crayon pieces (which always seem to be in over-supply) is to make stained-glass crayons. Remove any covering paper, place the pieces in a well-greased muffin tin (or line each muffin section with tin foil), and put in a 400° oven for a few minutes (or until melted). Remove from the oven and cool completely before removing from tin. If you mix the crayon colors, the circles will have a lovely stained-glass effect and are great fun to color with.

Peanut-Butter Bird Feeder

Spread peanut butter on each "leaf" of a pine cone. Roll in a dish of bird seed. Using a piece of yarn or wire, hang it from a tree.

Rainbow Celery

Place a cut stalk of celery with leaves still on it in a glass of water tinted with food coloring. Within an hour the color begins to show in the leaves. Slice one stalk in half part way up from the bottom and place each stem in separate glasses of differently colored water for a multicolored effect.

Chase the Pepper

You don't have to understand the scientific principle to be entertained by this magic trick.

Fill a pie plate (or small sink) with water. Shake pepper on the water. Take a piece of wet soap and dip it into the water. The pepper will run away from the soap. Now shake some sugar into the clear area and the pepper will run back.

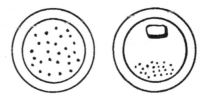

The Classic Rubber Egg

At least once in every childhood, one should experience the disgusting "rubber egg" experiment. Place an uncooked egg—in its shell—in a glass jar and pour white vinegar over it until covered. Leave for at least three days, then pour off vinegar. You will now have a yucky-to-the-touch but fascinating egg object.

Crystal Garden

4 tablespoons salt
4 tablespoons water
4 tablespoons ammonia

4 tablespoons liquid wash
   bluing

Mix ingredients. Pour over **several small pieces of charcoal or pieces of sponge in a bowl.** Put several drops of **different-colored inks** on various parts of it. Leave it undisturbed for a day. Crystals will cover it in an interesting formation, growing and spreading every day. It will be white where no ink was used. (The garden grows better in dry air than in humid air.)

How Does Your Garden Grow?

There are several easily grown items that may be of special wintertime delight for your child. He or she can do all the work.

A good functional container is a cut-down milk carton with potting soil and holes punched in the bottom for drainage. Or you may even want to use an egg-shell half. Three-quarters of an egg shell, decorated, makes a delightful pot. Better yet, the shell can be a "head" with green, growing "hair." Place "pot" in a sunny or well-lit window.

- **Avocados:** Though the avocado pit is a popular item to grow, it is not much fun for small children as germination is often very slow.

- **Cress:** Most types of cress are easy to grow and can even be added to salads a few weeks after planting.

- **Dried beans:** Roll a piece of paper towel and place in a clear glass. Put a bean (a lima bean, corn kernel, or other dried bean) between the paper and the side of the glass. Keep it moist. You can watch the seed send roots down and sprouts up.

- **Citrus seeds:** Place 4 or 5 seeds (orange, lemon, or grapefruit) in a container and cover with 1/2 inch of soil. Keep soil moist by gently covering with clear wrap until the seeds have germinated.

- **Sweet potatoes:** Place a large sweet potato in a shallow dish with enough water to cover it. Keep it half-covered in water as the days pass. It will grow a lovely vine for you. If you have no luck, try a new potato, since sweet potatoes are often treated to prevent growth.

- **Carrots:** Cut the green top from a carrot yourself. Place top few inches of the carrot root in water. Top will sprout again.

- **Grass seed or bird seed:** Place on a wet sponge in a shallow dish. A little water should always show above the sponge, so that you know it has not dried out. Your child can "mow the lawn" if he or she can handle a scissors.

Parent Potpourri
(Or, "I Wish I'd Thought of That!")

This final chapter is a collection of everything that didn't fit anyplace else. It contains many well-used ideas passed from "practicing" parents to other new parents—practical information collected in one place for your reference.

Busy Little People Make Spots

Some tried-and-true methods for removing those spots that are sure to show up as your child grows:

- **Stamped-on prices:** Remove from plastic items with alcohol or cleaning fluid. Labels usually come off with either peanut butter, baby oil, cooking oil, or hot vinegar.

- **Milk spots on upholstery or carpet:** Rub in baking soda and vacuum out. Baking soda will prevent staining and keep odor away. Other stains often disappear using window cleaner spray or just baby wipes.

- **Blood stains:** Rinse in cold water. Then soak in cold water with salt before washing as usual. Or let hydrogen peroxide bubble through the fabric to help release the stain before washing.

127

- **Urine on a rug:** This requires fast action. Mix a solution of 1/2 cup vinegar with 3/4 cup water. Apply small amounts on the stain. Give the solution a few minutes to work and then sponge from the outside to the center. Blot dry with a cloth. Keep the above solution on hand so that prompt action is possible. Another recommended solution is 1 tablespoon ammonia in 3/4 cup water. Use small amounts and blot out.

- **Marks on appliances and windows:** Clean without film or streaks with this solution. Mix 1/4 cup alcohol, 1 tablespoon white vinegar, and 1 tablespoon nonsudsy ammonia. Add enough hot water to make one quart.

With a baby:

- **Baby bottles and toys:** A few spoonfuls of baking soda in a quart of water cleans baby bottles and toys and freshens a diaper bag and plastic panties. Add baking soda to your diaper pail to prevent odor.

- **Baby's silver gifts:** To clean, rub a small amount of toothpaste over them with a damp cloth, then rinse clean.

- **After-meal mess:** After-meal "swabbing" is seldom appreciated by babies. You can ease the task by applying petroleum jelly or baby oil to your baby's chin and cheeks before a meal. Or when your little one is able, give him or her a damp washcloth (or a puppet washcloth) for a self-cleanup. If the washcloth is warm (or a soft baby washcloth), you'll probably meet with less resistance. Play peek-a-boo with a washcloth, cleaning a little off each time. Most (though not all) of the food will be removed and so will the hassle. You can also hold a small bowl of water on a highchair tray after a meal while your child plays with the water for a minute. Then all you need to do is wipe the clean hands dry! A dab of toothpaste spread over an upper-lip juice stain removes it quickly.

- **Highchair cleanup:** In warm weather, take it outside and hose it down. Otherwise, give it a shower in your shower.

With a toddler:

- **Crayon marks:** Remove from vinyl tile or linoleum with silver polish. To remove from woodwork, rub lightly with a dry, soap-filled steel-wool pad.

- **Dirty white socks:** Boil in water with a slice of lemon. Or let a load of them soak in hot water in your washing machine for a half hour using 1/2 cup automatic dishwasher detergent. If the socks are cotton, add 1 cup of chlorine bleach. If they're a blend, use a nonchlorine whitener.

- **Ball-point ink on fabrics:** Remove by spraying hair spray directly on surface and wiping away with warm, sudsy water. It's the alcohol in it that makes it work.

- **Bubble gum in the hair:** Peanut butter is a terrific remedy. (Then you're just stuck with washing out the peanut butter!) Milk chocolate and cold cream are also effective. To remove bubble gum on fabric, cover area with a piece of waxed paper and run a warm iron over the wax paper quickly, until the gum dissolves.

- **Stuffed toys:** Clean by rubbing with corn starch. Let stand briefly, then brush off.

- **Finger marks on wallpaper:** Rub chunks of soft, stale bread over wallpaper to remove.

- **Velcro losing its stick?:** Run a stiff toothbrush, a pen, or a fine-toothed metal comb through the rough, looped side.

Don't forget to keep those handy stain sticks around, in a diaper bag, your changing area, or near the washing machine. (*But remember, they're not for a little one to play with!*)

Now You Are an M.D.—Mother-on-Duty

Motherhood, you will quickly discover, is an on-the-job paramedic training program.

First, keep in mind that feeding schedules usually disappear during illness. Even a minor illness usually means that foods give way to liquids. Give your child plenty to drink, if the child is not vomiting. Your child's appetite will make up for the lost meals when good health returns.

129

Your doctor may recommend a clear-liquid diet. This includes Fruit Ice, Popsicles, frozen orange-juice-on-a-stick, Kool-Aid, clear broth, Jell-O, fruit punches, and soft drinks such as cola or ginger ale that have been allowed to go flat.

If your child won't drink the needed liquids, offer a straw when he or she is in a bathtub of clean water.

Fruit Ice is an excellent first-aid measure for cut lips and bumped mouths. It slows down bleeding and keeps swelling to a minimum, while getting your child's mind off the discomfort.

Fruit Ice

finely crushed ice
frozen juice concentrate, thawed

Place ice in a cup and pour juice over it. Drink or eat as a snow cone with a spoon.

First-Aid Tips

- Give a child liquid medicine in a nipple, an eye-dropper, or a syringe dispenser you can buy at the drugstore. (*Don't give medications in the dark.*)

- Honey and lemon juice make a good homemade cough syrup. (*Do not give to babies under one year old.*)

- A small plastic hair curler makes a good "cast" for a bruised finger. And a wooden pop stick can be used as a splint.

- An ice cube will help numb an area when you need to remove a splinter.

- Use a can of frozen juice or a bag of frozen vegetables as a quick, dripless compress. Or keep in your freezer a zip-sealed plastic bag filled with half water and half rubbing alcohol. It, too, will conform to different shapes. Refreeze and use as needed.

- When removing an adhesive bandage, rub it well first with baby oil to make it "ouchless."

- A pill is swallowed more easily in a teaspoon of applesauce.

- Give liquid vitamins during bath time to avoid stains on clothes.

- Treat a bee sting quickly with a paste of baking soda and water. Or use meat tenderizer and water. Ice can help numb the area.

- For diaper rash, cautiously use your hair dryer to dry a sore bottom between diaper changes. Fresh air, in any form, is the best treatment for a rampant rash. Solid vegetable shortening can be used as a diaper-rash ointment.

- Immediate treatment for a burn is cold water and/or ice. For a larger burn (including sunburn), cover area with a cold, wet towel.

- Keep warm compresses warm in a crock pot.

Illness Feeding Guideline

Sore Throat

Offer soothing suckers (such as lollipops, Popsicles, frozen orange-juice-on-a-stick), ice cream, and ice chips.

Fever

Give liquids in whatever form your child will take them. If your child won't drink large amounts, try small amounts at frequent intervals. Sometimes your child will drink more by going back to a bottle. Check with your doctor before you give aspirin or acetaminophen.

Vomiting

Forget food; wait as long as your child will let you to try small amounts of liquid. To assure a slow intake, let your child suck on an ice cube or on crushed ice. Continue to add small amounts of liquids in gradually increasing intervals until you are sure your child's stomach is settled. Appropriate liquids are decarbonated sodas, sweetened tea, and "Jell-O Water" (add one package Jell-O to one quart of water). Wait half a day before starting easy solids such as dry crackers. If vomiting recurs, start from the top. Check with your doctor if vomiting continues into a second day.

Diarrhea

Discontinue milk (including skim, boiled, or unboiled) until symptoms disappear. Serve appropriate liquids at room temperature: juices, decarbonated sodas, weak tea, "Jell-O Water" (in this case, one package Jell-O to one cup tap water), and carrot soup (make by mixing one jar of commercial strained carrots with one jar of water—it replaces fluids as well as lost minerals). Easy-binding solids are: mashed potatoes, rice cereal, Jell-O, dry toast, crackers, banana, and applesauce. Check with your doctor if your baby is under six months of age. Give Gatorade to older children to replace lost minerals as well as fluids. Easy to remember is the BRAT diet:

BRAT Diet

Bananas
Rice cereal
Applesauce
Toast

Serve small meals from this list every four hours to control diarrhea in young children.

Constipation

Serve lots of liquids! Water, diluted prune juice, noncitrus fruit juices, fruits, and yogurt are best. For children over one year of age, add a teaspoon of dark Karo syrup to milk, formula, or water. Avoid milk products, apples, bananas, rice, or gelatin, as they are binding.

Many well-meaning parents think a child is "constipated" if there is a bowel movement "only" every other day or every three days. But what is important is the child's individual, established pattern of bowel movements (or stools) and the ease of passing them. A normal frequency of stools can vary from several times a day to as infrequently as once a week, if there is no straining or discomfort. Small, very hard, dry, rock-like stools passed daily or very large, firm, bulky stools passed once a week—and which clog up the toilet—are both signs of constipation.

Back to Eating

Here are some ideas for coaxing an ailing child back to eating when his or her health returns.

- Offer snacks frequently to break boredom, supplement small appetites, and increase intake of fluids.
- Allow an "eat-where-you-want" policy.
- Try novelty eating utensils such as toothpicks.
- Serve foods in tiny portions in muffin tins or egg cartons.
- Place fruit juice in an insulated pitcher at bedside.
- Put soup in a mug.
- Make sandwich tacos and cookie-cutter sandwiches.
- Stage an indoor picnic on the floor.

Poisons— A Very Real Danger

Do you know the phone number of your poison-control center?

My poison center number is _____
The information needed by phone or at the hospital is the child's *age, weight, type and amount of poison ingested, and symptoms.*

Take the container with you to the phone and/or the hospital.

Poisons pose a very real danger to your child. Write your poison-control phone number down now—not later. Later may be too late. Call this number now to ask about "Mr. Yuk" stickers. The stickers can be affixed to household containers holding potential poisons.

The hand of the toddler can be quicker than the eye. Prevention is the best and the only cure. Do not store "poison" in low storage areas and remember that high, safe places are no longer safe when your child can climb. Lock up all your medicines. By doing so, you will convey the attitude of precaution. Poisons include household cleaners, paints, lotions, creams, polish, bleach, but especially aspirin! Don't get in the habit of treating medicine like candy, because it just might be eaten that way when you're not near.

Some plants are also poisonous. These include hyacinth and daffodil bulbs, dieffenbachia (all parts), caster bean (all parts), lily-of-the-valley (leaves and flowers), iris (rhizome), rhubarb (leaves, cooked or raw), wild cherries, jack-in-the-pulpit (all parts), and others. Acorns consumed in quantity can be poisonous; don't let your child chew on them.

Different poisons require different antidotes. Before doing anything, call your poison-control center. If the child is unconscious, call your local emergency number (911 in most locations).

In general, do **not** induce vomiting if the swallowed substance is a corrosive or petroleum product. Try to have the child drink water.

If the poison is a noncorrosive substance and if the child is conscious and not convulsing, give him or her a drink of water and then try to induce vomiting. Before you follow through on these suggestions, get medical advice. BUT REMEMBER TO CALL YOUR POISON-CONTROL CENTER FIRST.

Always keep syrup of ipecac on hand—a safe drug for inducing vomiting. But it should not be used without advice from a poison-control center, a hospital, or a doctor. It is inexpensive and available at all pharmacies without a prescription. If you already have this substance in your medicine cabinet, check the expiration date on the bottle.

Choking

If your child begins to choke but he or she can breathe (as indicated by coughing or speaking), do not do anything.

If the air passageway is indeed blocked, then three back blows properly administered can be effective, but the Heimlich maneuver has been shown to be the most effective treatment for airway obstruction in children.

To administer the Heimlich maneuver properly and know how to do it for children of different ages, take a local CPR course. It is important to administer it correctly and yet gently enough not to cause internal injuries to a child. Don't practice this at home on your children.

Traveling Tips—Eating En Route

Following these few suggestions about eating while traveling will help make your trips more enjoyable.

- Carry a plastic jug of sterile water to assure you of uniformity and sterility. Water varies greatly around the country and can cause problems for a baby.

- Fresh milk can be purchased everywhere, but do be sure that the container is sealed and states that it has been pasteurized. For the older baby on fresh milk, thorough cleaning of bottles and nipples is all that's required, since germs cannot multiply on clean, dry surfaces.

- Or if you prefer, put premeasured nonfat dry milk in a bottle. Add water as needed.

- Take along a wide-mouth thermos to keep baby's bottle warm. The ribbed portion of an old sock can fit over a bottle to give it better insulation and make it easier for a child to hold.

- When traveling by plane, let your baby drink from a bottle during takeoffs and landings. This will relieve the pressure in the ears of a child too young to understand the technique of swallowing. An older child can suck on a lollipop or chew gum.

- Bring along edibles that are easy on the tummy, such as crackers, cheese, fresh fruit, juices, and toast with peanut butter. Bagels are good too, and less crumby.

- Don't forget a packet of moistened wipes or a damp wash-cloth in a plastic bag.

- Throw leftovers away unless you have a cooler with you.

- Use a covered cake pan to hold paper, washable markers, colored pencils and crayons (not in hot weather) for car traveling entertainment.

- Arrive at a restaurant before the crowds. This will usually give you the extra service you need.

Some Final Pass-Along Ideas

Here are some of the best "practical parenting" tips. (For over 1500 more, see my *Practical Parenting Tips,* Meadowbrook Press.)

- When your child becomes an "artist," use kitchen magnets instead of tape to affix the pictures to your refrigerator.

- Recycle baby-food jars. Use in your tool box; for rock collections; for freezing small quantities of food; in a muffin tin to hold paints without spilling; as a small bank; as spice jars; as decorated party favors filled with treats.

- A collection of baby-food jar-tops in a plastic container is a great treat for an eight-month-old.

- When your child reaches the age when he or she doesn't want foods "touching" on a dinner plate, try compartmentalized plates.

- Nonskid appliqués or strips made for the bathtub are ideal for the highchair to keep baby from sliding down in the seat.

- If you can spare a bottom drawer in the kitchen, turn it into a toy drawer. It is handy both for toy pickups and for fast distractions!

- If your child objects to a bib, a colorful bandanna scarf will serve as one for your "cowboy" or "cowgirl."

And, *finally,* some food for thought from an anonymous author:

How To Bake a Cake

Light oven. Get out bowl, spoons, and ingredients. Grease pan. Crack nuts. Remove 18 blocks and 7 toy autos from kitchen table. Measure 2 cups of flour. Remove Kelly's hands from flour. Wash flour off. Measure 1 more cup of flour to replace flour on floor. Put flour, baking powder, and salt in a sifter. Get dustpan to brush up pieces of bowl Kelly knocked to floor. Get another bowl. Answer phone. Return. Take out greased pan. Remove pinch of salt from pan. Look for Kelly. Get another pan and grease it. Answer phone. Return to kitchen and find Kelly. Remove grimy hands from bowl. Wash off shortening. Take greased pan and find 1/4 inch of nutshells in it. Head for Kelly who flees, knocking bowl off table. Wash kitchen floor, wash table, wash walls, wash dishes, wash Kelly.

Call bakery.

Lie down.

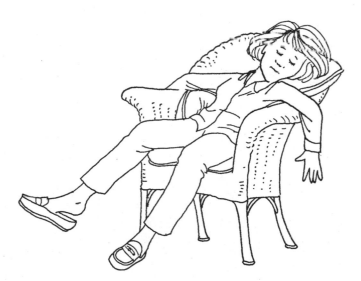

INDEX

FOOD EQUIVALENTS FOR MILK

1 cup buttermilk	=	1 cup milk
1 cup yogurt	=	1 cup milk
1/2 cup ice cream	=	1/4 cup milk
1/2 cup ice milk	=	1/3 cup milk
1 cup baked custard	=	1 cup milk
1 ounce (slice) Swiss cheese	=	1 cup milk
1 slice American processed cheese	=	1/2 cup milk
1-inch-cube cheddar cheese	=	1/2 cup milk
1 cup cottage cheese (creamed)	=	1/3 cup milk
2 tablespoons cream cheese	=	1 tablespoon milk

MILK SUBSTITUTES

Baking and run out of milk or cream? Remember that:

If the recipe calls for:	You can substitute:
1 cup coffee cream	3 tablespoons butter plus 7/8 cup milk
1 cup heavy cream	1/3 cup butter plus 3/4 cup milk
1 cup whole milk	1 cup reconstituted nonfat dry milk plus 2-1/2 teaspoons butter or margarine or 1/2 cup evaporated milk plus 1/2 cup water
1 cup buttermilk or juice	1 tablespoon vinegar or lemon juice plus enough sweet milk to make 1 cup (let stand 5 minutes before using)

TO USE HONEY INSTEAD OF SUGAR WHEN BAKING

- Use 2/3 cup of honey for each cup of sugar called for.
- For each cup of honey that you use, deduct about 3 tablespoons of liquid for the recipe. (This does not apply to yeast bread.) In baked goods, add 1/2 teaspoon soda for every cup substituted.
- Reduce oven temperature by about 25 degrees and bake a little longer, as honey tends to make baked goods brown faster.

  To use honey instead of brown sugar, use some molasses with the honey.

SIZE OF CAN

8 ounces	=	1 cup
9 ounces	=	No. 1 flat or 1 cup
16 ounces	=	No. 1 tall or 2 cups
16 ounces	=	No. 303
12 ounces	=	No. 2 vacuum or 1-3/4 cups
20 ounces (18 fluid)	=	No. 2 or 2-1/2 cups
28 ounces	=	No. 2-1/2 or 3-1/2 cups
46 ounces	=	No. 3 cylinder or 5-3/4 cups
6 lbs. 10 ounces	=	No. 10 or 13 cups

MEASURE FOR MEASURE

1 pound flour	=	4 cups
1 stick or		
1/4 pound butter	=	1/2 cup
1 square chocolate	=	1 ounce
14 squares graham crackers	=	1 cup fine crumbs
1-1/2 slices bread	=	1 cup soft crumbs
4 ounces macaroni		
(1-1/4 cups)	=	2-1/4 cups cooked
4 ounces noodles		
(1-1/2–2 cups)	=	2 cups cooked
1 cup long grain rice	=	3–4 cups cooked
juice of one lemon	=	3 tablespoons
grated peel of 1 lemon	=	1 teaspoon
juice of one orange	=	1/3 cup
grated peel of 1 orange	=	2 teaspoons
1 medium apple, chopped	=	1 cup
1 medium banana, mashed	=	1/3 cup
1 pound American cheese		
(shredded)	=	4 cups
1 pound raisins	=	3-1/2 cups
1 pound carrots	=	4 medium or 6 small
		3 cups shredded
		2-1/2 cups diced
1 cup milk	=	1/2 cup evaporated milk plus 1/2 cup water OR 1/3 cup dry milk plus one cup water
1 cup sour milk	=	1 teaspoon vinegar or lemon juice plus fresh milk to make 1 cup (let stand 5 minutes before using)

WEIGHTS AND MEASURES

3 teaspoons	=	1 tablespoon
4 tablespoons	=	1/4 cup
8 tablespoons	=	1/2 cup
16 tablespoons	=	1 cup
1 cup	=	8 ounces
1 cup	=	1/2 pint
2 cups	=	1 pint
2 pints	=	1 quart
4 cups	=	1 quart
4 quarts	=	1 gallon

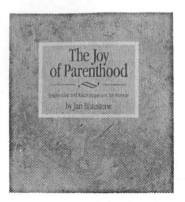

The Joy of Parenthood
by Jan Blaustone

This book contains over a hundred pages of warm and inspirational "nuggets" of wisdom to help prepare parents for the pleasures and challenges ahead. Twenty-four touching black-and-white photos help convey the joy of parenthood and make this a delightful book to give or receive.

"An inspiring tribute to the joy of being a parent."
—H. Jackson Brown, Jr., author of *Life's Little Instruction Book*
Order #3500

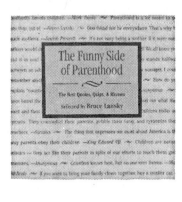

The Funny Side of Parenthood
selected by Bruce Lansky

A treasury of the most outrageous and clever things ever said about raising children by comedians and humorists including Roseanne Arnold, Erma Bombeck, Bill Cosby, Dave Barry, Mark Twain, and Fran Lebowitz. An excellent gift for any parent—anytime.
Order # 4015

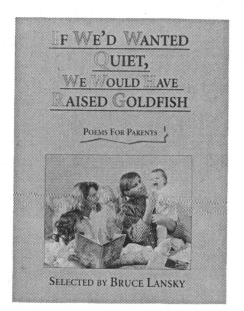

If We'd Wanted Quiet,
We Would Have Raised Goldfish
selected by Bruce Lansky

Get ready for an emotional experience. This collection of poems about having and raising children will move you to laughter or tears, even if you haven't read a poem since you were in school.

Selected for their ability to evoke feelings every parent has had in words every parent can understand, the poems in this book cover the entire range of parenting experience from conception to caring for your aging parents. They will linger in your memory long after you've read them.

Open this book and read the first poem you see. Don't be surprised when you turn the page and keep reading—and then find yourself wanting to share this book with others.

Order #3505

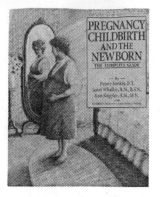

Pregnancy, Childbirth, and the Newborn
by Simkin, Whalley, and Keppler

The most complete and doctor-recommended childbirth guide available, it explains and shows (with 150 photos and illustrations, and 45 charts) how to prepare yourself for a healthy, positive birth experience. It covers nutrition, exercise, labor comfort measures, anesthesia choices, birth, breastfeeding, and new baby care. Childbirth experts call the book, created by the Childbirth Education Association of Seattle, their "bible."
Order #1169

First-Year Baby Care
edited by Paula Kelly, M.D.

Since babies don't come with an "owner's manual," we created one to help you anticipate and handle your new baby's basic needs without worry. This helpful handbook covers feeding, bathing, first aid, health, childproofing, and sleeping (good luck!). Newly revised, this book gives new parents the techniques and confidence they need.
Order #1119

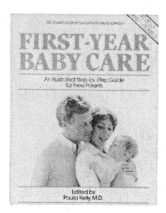

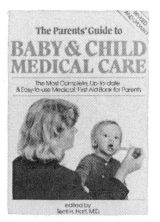

The Parents' Guide to Baby & Child Medical Care
edited by Terril Hart, M.D.

Every first-aid or medical problem your child suffers seems like an emergency. That's why you need this easy-to-read-and-use source of medical information at your fingertips. Newly revised, this book provides illustrated step-by-step instructions that show you what to do and tell you when to call your doctor. Its visual approach makes the book much easier to use than Dr. Spock's.
Order #1159

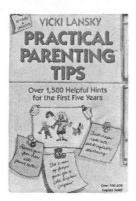

Practical Parenting Tips
by Vicki Lanksy

Here's the #1-selling collection of helpful hints for parents of babies and small children. It contains 1001 parent-tested tips for dealing with diaper rash, nighttime crying, toilet training, temper tantrums, and traveling with tots. It will help you save trouble, time, and money.

Order #1180

Discipline without Shouting or Spanking
by Jerry Wyckoff, Ph.D., and Barbara C. Unell

Do you know all the theories about child rearing but still have trouble coping with some of your child's misbehavior? You'll love this book! It covers the 30 most common forms of misbehavior from whining, clinging, and talking back to not eating, resisting bedtime, and temper tantrums. You'll find clear, practical advice on what to do, what not to do, and how to prevent each problem from recurring.

Order #1079

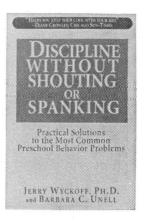

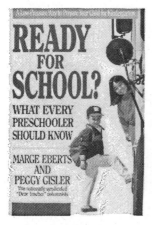

Ready for School?
by Marge Eberts and Peggy Gisler

A recent survey of kindergarten teachers warns: Don't force-feed reading and math to your preschooler! This practical book offers a low-pressure way to prepare your child for kindergarten that really works. It tells you how to help your child learn the basic skills required for kindergarten without turning into a "teacher." Eberts and Gisler are former teachers who write "Dear Teacher," a nationally syndicated newspaper column. They show how much fun it can be to share learning activities with your preschooler.

Order #1360

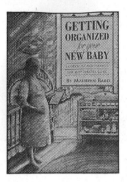

Getting Organized for Your New Baby
by Maureen Bard

Here's the fastest way to get organized for pregnancy, childbirth, and new baby care. Busy expectant parents love the checklists, forms, schedules, charts, and hints in this book because they make getting ready so much easier.

Order #1229

The Best Baby Name Book in the Whole Wide World
by Bruce Lansky

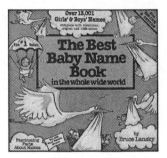

This really is the best baby name book! Over 13,000 names, complete with derivations and meanings—more contemporary names than any other book. Other helpful features include expert advice on how to pick an appropriate name, legal information about names, plus the 200 most popular names. No wonder it's the best-selling baby name book in the U.S. and Canada.

Order #1029

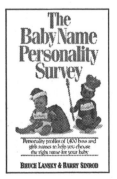

The Baby Name Personality Survey
by Bruce Lansky & Barry Sinrod

This fascinating book is based on a national survey of 75,000 parents—the largest name research project ever. It reveals the images and stereotypes associated with 1,400 popular and unusual names. Find out what other people think of the names you're considering before you make a decision that will last a lifetime.

Order #1270

Dads Say the Dumbest Things!

by Bruce Lansky and Ken Jones

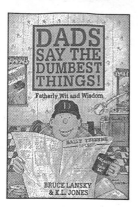

Lansky and Jones have collected all the greatest lines dads have ever used to get kids to stop fighting in the car, feed the pet, turn off the TV while doing their homework, and get home before curfew from a date. It includes such winners as: "What do you want a pet for—you've got a sister" and "When I said 'feed the goldfish,' I didn't mean feed them to the cat." A fun gift for dad.

Order #4220

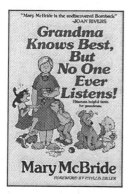

Moms Say the Funniest Things!

by Bruce Lansky

A collection of all the greatest lines moms have ever used to deal with "emergencies" like getting the kids out of bed, cleaned, dressed, to school, to the dinner table, undressed, and back to bed. Includes such all-time winners as: "Put on clean underwear—you never know when you'll be in an accident" and "If God had wanted you to fool around, He would have written 'Ten Suggestions.'"

Order #4280

Grandma Knows Best, But No One Ever Listens

by Mary McBride

Advice for new grandmas on how to
- Show baby photos to anyone at any time
- Get out of babysitting ... or if stuck, to housebreak the kids before they wreck the house
- Advise the daughter-in-law without being banned from her home

The perfect gift for grandma, it's "harder to put down than a new grandchild."
—Phyllis Diller

Order #4009

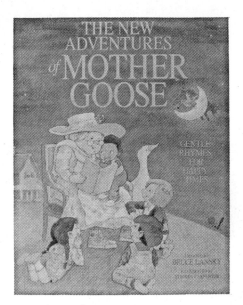

The New Adventures
of Mother Goose

created by Bruce Lansky
illustrated by Stephen Carpenter

Bruce Lansky and illustrator Stephen Carpenter have teamed up
to create all-new, funny, updated-for-the-'90s sequels to favorite
Mother Goose rhymes. The delightful new adventures are non-
sexist, nonviolent, and more modern. Every twist on the
traditional rhymes surprises and delights children, parents, and
grand-parents alike. A must-have book for every home with
young children.
Order #2420

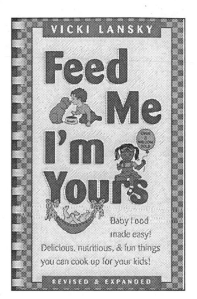

Feed Me! I'm Yours

by Vicki Lansky

The best-selling guide to making fresh, pure baby foods at home; over 200 recipes; lists of finger, fun, and birthday foods.
Order #1109

Free Catalog of Books by Vicki Lansky

For a free catalog of more than twenty books for parents and children by Vicki Lansky,

call: 1-800-255-3379

or write: Practical Parenting
Dept. PPT
18326 Minnetonka Blvd.
Deephaven, MN 55391

Order Form

Qty.	Title	Author	Order No.	Unit Cost	Total
	10,000 Baby Names	Lansky, B.	1210	$3.50	
	35,000+ Baby Names	Lansky, B.	1225	$5.95	
	Baby & Child Emergency First-Aid	Einzig, M.	1381	$8.00	
	Baby & Child Medical Care	Hart, T.	1159	$8.00	
	Baby Name Personality Survey	Lansky/Sinrod	1270	$8.00	
	Best Baby Name Book	Lansky, B.	1029	$5.00	
	Dads Say the Dumbest Things!	Lansky/Jones	4220	$6.00	
	Discipline w/o Shouting or Spanking	Wyckoff/Unell	1079	$6.00	
	Feed Me! I'm Yours	Lansky, V.	1109	$9.00	
	First-Year Baby Care	Kelly, P.	1119	$7.00	
	Free Stuff For Kids	F.S. Editors	2190	$5.00	
	Funny Side of Parenthood	Lansky, B.	4015	$6.00	
	Gentle Discipline	Lighter, D.	1085	$6.00	
	Getting Organized for Your Baby	Bard, M.	1229	$9.00	
	Grandma Knows Best	McBride, M.	4009	$6.00	
	Happy Helpful Grandma Guide	Spirson, L.	1290	$8.00	
	If We'd Wanted Quiet/Poems for Parents	Lansky, B.	3505	$12.00	
	Joy of Parenthood	Blaustone, J.	3500	$6.00	
	Moms Say the Funniest Things!	Lansky, B.	4280	$6.00	
	New Adventures of Mother Goose	Lansky, B.	2420	$15.00	
	Practical Parenting Tips	Lansky, V.	1180	$8.00	
	Pregnancy, Childbirth, and the Newborn	Simkin, Whalley, Keppler	1169	$12.00	
				Subtotal	
			Shipping and Handling (see below)		
			MN residents add 6.5% sales tax		
				Total	

YES, please send me the books indicated above. Add $2.00 shipping and handling for the first book and $.50 for each additional book. Add $2.50 to total for books shipped to Canada. Overseas postage will be billed. Allow up to 4 weeks for delivery. Send check or money order payable to Meadowbrook Press. No cash or C.O.D.'s please. Prices subject to change without notice.
Quantity discounts available upon request.

Send book(s) to:

Name_____

Address_____

City _____State _____ Zip_____

Telephone (_____) _____

Payment via:

☐ Check or money order payable to Meadowbrook (No cash or C.O.D., please.)
  Amount enclosed $ _____

☐ Visa (for orders over $10.00 only.)

☐ MasterCard (for orders over $10.00 only.)

Account # _____

Signature _____ Exp. Date_____

You can also phone us for orders of $10.00 or more at 1-800-338-2232.

A **Free** Meadowbrook Press catalog is available upon request.

Mail to: Meadowbrook, Inc.
18318 Minnetonka Boulevard, Deephaven, Minnesota 55391
(612) 473-5400   Toll-Free 1-800-338-2232   Fax (612) 475-0736